The Singing Forest

A Journey Through Lyme Disease

© 2006 by PJ Langhoff

The Singing Forest, A Journey Through Lyme Disease

A print-on-demand publication

ISBN 978-1-4116-9529-0

The text of this book is 13 point Times New Roman, and 18 point Skia. I have enlarged it wherever possible, for those with Lyme who find it difficult to read small print.

For more information, please write the author at:
PJ Langhoff, PO Box 444, Hustisford, Wisconsin, 53034 • U.S.A. Please visit www.LymeLeague.com, www.Sewill.org and other important Lyme Links located at the end of this book.

Printed in the United States of America

I dedicate this book to every person
who has ever been, or will be touched by
Lyme disease and its co-infections.

You are *not* alone.

❖

A special thanks to Dr. James L. Schaller,
whose incredible insight and experience
with Lyme disease in his own family
possessed him to read "The Forgotten" and
recognize the powerful emotions expressed there.
I am humbly grateful to you and for your efforts
on behalf of Lyme patients everywhere.

❖

And to Dr. Charles Ray Jones,
an intelligent, prominent pediatric Lyme specialist,
I would allow my children to be treated by you,
anywhere, and anytime. You are an absolute treasure.

❖

As I sat upon the judgement's stand,
I witnessed the dawning of a new process.
It came from within, a golden light,
illuminating ignorance with new understanding.
And filled my heart with hope for the future,
of promises kept, an end to innocent suffering.
That hope was my strength; the knowledge of righteous grace.
that in the end, I had done the *right* thing,
and *that* grace can never be removed.

– *The author*

❖ TABLE OF CONTENTS ❖

"Defending the truth is not something
one does out of a sense of duty
or to allay guilt complexes, but is a reward in itself."

— *Peter Bechmann*

❖The Disclaimer❖

Since people are so hyped up in this day and age about lawsuits and personal responsibility, I feel it sad but nevertheless important to include a disclaimer in this book. For those inclined to refuse their own personal responsibility and who seek to blame others for the outcome of their decisions or lack thereof based upon anything implied, said, not said, inferred or otherwise described as either for or against, read this book at your own risk, you are wholly responsible for yourself, not I.

For those other entities who might try to stifle my freedom of speech, remember that our forefathers won that right through the sacrifice of their blood and lives to produce this great nation. There are many actively defending those rights as I write this, and to them I say "thank you". I am humbly and forever grateful for your service and sacrifice.

I am *not* a medical doctor. I do not have a medical degree. I *do* have some college credit in various subjects that I never had the opportunity to form into a formal degree. In this book, although I will give my opinion about medical and legal issues, I have no authority to do so from any standpoint except as a patient of this insidious illness. The contents of this book are my personal opinion. As one doctor has (quite sadly), previously said to me, "What do you know, you're just the patient?"

For those who might argue that I am attempting to exploit my own and my family's experiences, I must vehemently deny that accusation. The events portrayed in this book, while incredibly private, as a whole paint an accurate picture of the long-range damage thrust upon this family, caused by the ignorance and denial surrounding Lyme disease.

In the interests of raising greater awareness of Lyme and its far-reaching consequences, the value that comes from telling this story, in my opinion, far surpasses the need for silence, and perhaps even supercedes any authority projected by those who might try to prevent my doing so.

It is only through listening to the patients who have to deal with Lyme or any disease on a daily basis, that anyone, no matter how well-educated, will learn the lessons that disease teaches, and ultimately lead to its proper treatment; and one day, a cure.

In medicine, the doctor has the difficult responsibility to listen to their patient and objectively seek a solution to their condition. In Lyme disease, this is very hard to do, especially when office visits have replaced the house call, malpractice lawsuits abound, and physicians have pressures from agencies that are perhaps profit-driven or that track their diagnostic habits to be scrutinized, analyzed and publicized as they see fit. Making it even more challenging are the varying symptoms, the lack of definitive testing and large array of misinformation that is currently available about Lyme disease.

All doctors are not exempt from having treated their patients with less than kind regards. Some treat their patients as if they are somehow less intelligent than the doctor himself. Others tell the patient that their illness is all in their head, and it is partly those individuals for whom I am writing this book.

One particular physician told me as I visited him 4 years before I had an accurate diagnosis of Lyme disease, "I'm not going to hold your hand every time you think there is something wrong with you." To him and others like him, I say, "why can't you? You are so much more than a doctor when you *hold* my hand. Together we walk through this illness, with you learning from me, and me receiving compassionate care so that I can become well. I live in my body, you know how it functions. Together we can achieve wellness". A house divided falls; a house united stands strong.

Furthermore, those that would attempt to dismiss disease of any kind in order to prevent panic, control costs, and limit access to information are indeed fostering the very extinction of mankind; one disease, and one human being, at a time.

When physicians are put upon the witness stand to defend the very oath they took when becoming a physician, it is a tragedy. When Lyme victims are persecuted in a court of law for their disease; or workers forced out of their jobs because they are ill, that is pure discrimination of the very worst kind.

And in my opinion, by allowing insurance companies, medical boards, pharmaceutical corporations and others to set criteria for who can be diagnosed, cured, given benefits, and/or receive treatment in order to control costs, or to follow some hidden agenda, the entire system of managed health care to me, has somehow managed to make itself obsolete.

I wonder sometimes how there manage to be any doctors remaining and willing to practice. To those that do remain, I urge you to consider the face of Lyme disease as told by the one who knows it best, its victim, and become more educated within this unique arena.

To legislators, I invite you to vote to change the laws to protect the patients as well as their physicians, so that together we can work as a team. Doctors can then effectively function without fear of reprisal as well as uphold the commitment they so purposely were sworn to perform.

Thank you for reading this book. I am just a small voice out of thousands with Lyme; and yet, I am not alone. We are banding together to make our voices heard. *Together we truly grow stronger.* ❖

"How many will listen
to the truth when you tell them?"

– *Old Yiddish Proverb*

❖ Foreword ❖

Not long ago I came across a poem sent by a very wise, mature political activist. She is a tough and seasoned person with a strong business orientation, who really has seen it all. I was surprised to see the excitement in her email about a poem.

Then I read the poem. After the first few lines of the poem by PJ Langhoff, I started to find my eyes dilating and my brain expanding. My entire being was inhaling in a way that only the mystics strive to describe. I had had this experience before in the presence of very rare and very special people–individuals with a very rare prophetic genius.

I suppose that is how it felt to those who first heard the Rev. Martin Luther King as he was flowering into his calling. Or those who listened to Mother Teresa speak about "human dignity in the weak who manifest the image of God," as she walked among those who seemingly least displayed it in their utter weakness.

As I read the poem I started to shudder and shake, not with revulsion, but with the sense I was witnessing the birth of someone who possessed many rare gifts, which fused, and became a spokesperson for millions. PJ Langhoff is that person.

In the same way I could not stop reading her poem, I believe in time, many will not be able to pull away from her. In a time of much "data" and mere information, she offers a mixture of experience, wisdom, passion and clarity that only a prophetess can offer.

I have lived in areas in which walking to the mailbox through a well groomed lawn is a risk. Lyme disease and its many co-infections is something I understand personally, due to my experience with my immediate and distant family and friends. Loved ones with boundless energy, over years, could not rise from a chair. Others became irritable and excessively sensitive, and they struggled to treat their children, spouse, friends and coworkers with civility. Others developed various illnesses and psychiatric trouble. Many lost their advanced cognitive edge and struggled to hide their fogginess. A couple drinks made them into different creatures—strangers to those who loved them and knew them.

My son's were each told they were fine by well meaning pediatricians. One son had a single very specific positive Western blot band, which simply means he had antibodies to a protein only found in those exposed to Lyme disease. My treasured child decayed over half a decade, as physician after physician offered useless information. Even respected academic and Ivy League centers mocked and actually despised me for suggesting he should be considered for Lyme. I simply had no idea what was wrong, and was trying to keep an open and curious mind.

Finally, after he could no longer function reasonably in school, I did for my son what I had done for so many in my medical practice. I fired all of his useless narrow thinking physicians, and I decided to find his cure. Of course, while I had done this with many illnesses before for my patients, I knew nothing about tick-borne illness, because my infectious disease mentors knew virtually nothing about it—though they acted like they could give God some lessons. It is no surprise to me that a passionate and motivated housewife discovered modern Lyme disease, in a flood of local children in the backyards of so many sleepy Ivy League schools.

My rejection of the reflexive and impulsive "wisdom" of five-minute pediatric evaluations is not unique to me. By the time my family was riddled with various tick borne infections, many tens of thousands of patients throughout the USA, had come to the conclusion that mainstream medicine was repeating its common error. They had fogged out on early HIV/AIDS information, they had ignored and mocked the idea of an infectious cause of stomach ulcers, and they had mocked the merits of essential nutrients while exclusively embracing drug company grants and ideology. Having published on both the usefulness of medications and nutrition, I felt I was in a good position to criticize.

But when my son's SPECT Scan came back with 70% of his brain inflamed with infection from Lyme, and higher quality lab testing showed clear and diffuse Lyme disease proteins throughout his blood, I was not able to calmly criticize. My level of hatred was so intense, that I was unable to speak. "This is not possible." I thought. "How can so many academic centers miss this for so many years as this infection ate my son's body away?"

I had believed in the merits of education, and had valued the notion of the specialist and the expert, but I was seeing my son slowly die in the name of these false cults. All the years of visits to experts who were certain of nothing except that "he did not have Lyme disease," came flying through my mind in image after image, as if I was dying. And I was dying, because to me, being a father was my deepest joy and deepest fear. The notion of losing a child as both my beloved grandparents had done was my greatest fear, and it was happening. His school was worthless, and in the simplistic psychology of the 1950's, the teachers and administration, tried to "help us" with our parenting. My wife and I listened to them gauge us with their titanic ignorance, and finally I explained to the principle of one old leaky moldy private school the magnitude of his ignorance. He was not happy. And I was beyond fed up listening to clique masters with their simplistic answers. Could school staff really be this utterly ignorant and useless? Again, I saw that a belief in the wisdom of schools is often misplaced. We successfully home schooled him for a year.

Another of my dear children was then found to have four Tick-borne infections, including the malaria-like Babesia. This infection does not respond to the same medications used for Lyme, and is one reason some Lyme patients died in past decades.

Of course we tried to explain these medical issues to their physicians, school, and our friends, but they simply listened with glazed eyes. Indeed, some of these NE USA residents clearly had signs of psychiatric and cognitive Lyme disease themselves, but the first thing to go is insight, so we were talking to the walking dead or to those who covet simplicity over reality.

Slowly, it became clear that many of my extended family members had Lyme and their symptoms were as unique as their DNA. Some had eccentric weight gain, others had trouble finishing a task, another was suddenly struggling with addictions, and another had decreased memory and was rigid. Another had joint and muscle aches that they attributed to "old age." Nonsense.

My family tried to follow the principles of some outspoken Ivy League Lyme "experts" and the leading infection society. Both claimed Lyme disease was magically killed in 30 days. You understand they did not suggest treating 29 days or 31 days, but 30 days exactly. They never seemed to say what one should do with co-infections, perhaps since they rarely tested for them.

I read their flawed studies and watched my children struggle with the absence of improvement, and finally turned to those who actually treated Lyme, instead of magically and sometimes fatally just wishing it away.

It was at this time that I met dozens of physicians involved with ILADS, a collection of physicians and other health care workers who were committed to advanced, reasonable and complete Lyme disease treatment. They had all seen the status quo treatments, and seen them kill people. So their position was to treat Lyme until the signs and symptoms were gone. It is hard to imagine that this is seen as either controversial or insightful—treat until a return to baseline health. That this is actually debated is unfathomable. You see too many anti-clinicians caught with Ivy around their neck, long-term antibiotics for a zit is fine, but using it to relieve and improve chronic Lyme symptoms, to them, is an abomination.

One physician who had treated 9,000 children with Tick-borne infections was in the backyard of Yale. His name was Charles Ray Jones. He was a pediatrician who had walked with Dr. Martin

Luther King in the early days, but then he turned his efforts toward medicine and pediatric cancer. After many discoveries and successes with cancer treatment, in the 60's, he slowly started to treat various Tick-borne infections. No one in the USA or the world has his decades of experience in pediatric tick-borne infections, and that experience helped to save the lives of my children.

And yet, despite his decades of sacrifice and service, he currently has to explain to the Connecticut state medical board and their "experts," who have a fraction of his experience, why he treated a child in another state who was found to be positive for Lyme disease on his lab tests without seeing her. It seems no one on the board has met a physician with a six month waiting list who works 12 hour days even when 78 years old and crippled? So because he decided to "do no harm" and prescribe an antibiotic to a sick symptomatic child on his six-month waiting list, he has to face a medical board with virtually no understanding or experience in pediatric Lyme disease.

Over the years, we have followed the advice of Dr. Jones and others in ILADS, and we have spent hundreds of thousands of dollars in the treatment of our immediate family, our wider families, friends from all over the USA who became infected, and to strangers who have received free care and had bills forgiven since they could not afford medical care or medication.

Currently, my children are largely recovered and enjoying a life without fatigue, sadness, memory trouble and aches. I am providing ongoing treatment since they are not fully cured. I am also working to help restore organs that may have been weakened by their undiagnosed infections. One of my best friends died quite suddenly of suspected Lyme disease, so I work to strengthen their bodies, so we will not be faced with their surprise deaths, something that is not rare in the Lyme community.

As a research and clinical physician, I treat patients from all over the USA who have been unable to find a cure for their illness.

Most have been to between five and forty smart and experienced physicians before me. Unfortunately, due to a lack of understanding from their sincere physicians, some of these individuals are ill from tick-borne infection like Lyme, and the routine labs used to test for it are of such poor and inferior quality, that even patients with the rare bulls-eye rash come up negative after one or more months. In other words, after the body has had plenty of time to make Lyme antibodies.

Most physicians do not realize that Lyme is present in every part of the United States, and that routine cheap labs only detect a limited number of Lyme strains. I often see individuals whose Lyme has been missed and who suffer with seizures, strokes, "ALS," embolisms, tics, mania, migraines, MS, autism, and heart damage. Sometimes I offer information to ill individuals and other physicians and they react with disdain to my gift. "They are too far-gone," some might say. I hope not. But many people have lost their ability to have insight into their own body and brain changes. Some are too lost because Lyme has affected their mind and they cannot consider other opinions. Lets hope those you love are not too far-gone.

I hope you are not too far-gone. I hope you can open your mind and heart to the exceptional material offered by one of medicine's new lay prophets. I offer this book to you with my strongest endorsements, knowing that this is important and well-written information that will empower and strongly encourage many people. You will also see that you are not crazy. *You are not alone.*   ❖

James Schaller, MD, MAR
Tampa and Naples, Florida
www.personalconsult.com

❖ Did You Know? ❖

The most common carrier of Lyme disease and co-infections is the tick. The tick is an arachnid, and like spiders, has a jointed body, limbs and eight legs. The most common hosts for ticks are white-footed mice, deer, birds and small animals.

Lyme Disease is the most common vector-borne disease in North America and Europe.

There are over 300 different genotypes of Borrelia burgdorferi (Bb), the spirochete that transmits Lyme disease to humans.

Ticks also transmit a host of other diseases when they bite. Some of these are: Ehrlichiosis, Babesiosis, Bartonella, Tularemia, Q-Fever, Mycoplasma, Anaplasma Phagocytophila, Tick-borne Encephalitis, Relapsing Fever, Rocky Mountain Spotted Fever, and many others.

The CDC (Centers for Disease Control) reported 166,868 cases of Lyme disease in the United States between the years of 1994-2003.

Most experts agree that the numbers are probably underreported by a factor of 10, and rapidly growing, with approximately 20,000 reported cases annually (but actual numbers are probably closer to 200,000).

Lyme has been reported in 49 out of 50 of the United States, and in Canada, Europe and other countries.

The best way to eliminate Lyme disease is through education and prevention. Short of that, proper diagnosis and treatment are *absolutely essential.*   ❖

"A doctor can always bury his mistakes,
but an architect can only tell his clients to plant vines."

– Frank Lloyd Wright

Chapter 1

First Things First

¹In the United States, Lyme disease, caused by the spirochete Borrelia burgdorferi (Bb), is reported approximately *eight times more often* than West Nile Virus. Despite this fact, funding is currently being set aside in a disproportionately larger amount to prevent and treat the West Nile virus than it is for Lyme disease.

In 2004, 19,804 cases of Lyme disease were reported by the Centers for Disease Control (CDC). The CDC provided approximately $5.6 million dollars for the prevention and treatment of Lyme disease, and the National Institutes of Health (NIH) contributed about $28 million dollars for this purpose.

For West Nile virus however, the number of cases reported that same year by the CDC was a mere 2,539. Nevertheless, the CDC spent a significantly higher amount of its funding, (nearly six times as much as on Lyme), or $34.6 million dollars, while the NIH contributed a whopping $43 million dollars to this cause; nearly doubling what it spent on Lyme.

After reviewing the aforementioned facts, as a Lyme patient, I would have to ask the obvious question; why is so much money being spent on the West Nile virus when there are so many Lyme patients; approximately eight times the number of West Nile cases?

According to a study published in 1993 by *Contingencies,* the long-range cost to society as a whole for Lyme disease was about $1 billion dollars annually. Since the number of Lyme disease cases has nearly doubled since that time, the costs are easily $2 billion dollars or more per year. The average costs of diagnosis, treatment and lost wages runs approximately $62,000 per year, per person. Many with Lyme are living on the verge of, or have already filed, bankruptcy.

Despite the growing incidence of Lyme disease and the high economic factors involved in dealing with it, patients are finding the diagnosis and treatment of their Lyme disease, increasingly more difficult to obtain. Many patients average 2-4 years and see over 20 doctors before they are diagnosed and/or treated for Lyme. It took 12-1/2 years for this author to obtain a diagnosis for herself and her two children. I have long since lost count of how many doctors we have seen, probably somewhere nearing 100. My personal medical records measure 10 inches high, and that does not even represent all of them.

The following excerpts were taken verbatim from the Centers for Disease Control and other web sites, in April of 2006. Items appearing in italics and brackets [ ] are the author's comments, and were not part of the published materials.

[2]**How are cases [of Lyme] reported to CDC?**

As with most other diseases, reporting requirements for Lyme disease are determined by state laws or regulations. In most states, Lyme disease cases are reported by licensed health care providers, diagnostic laboratories, or hospitals. States and the District of Columbia share their data with CDC, which compiles and publishes the information for the Nation.

[Note the state-level determination for reporting Lyme, varies between states. Licensed healthcare providers also complete a form when reporting, that merely takes into account where Lyme was first diagnosed, and not necessarily where it was contracted; often unknown.]

Are more recent numbers available?

Cases of Lyme disease and other reportable conditions are published each week in the MMWR. However, these weekly numbers are provisional and often change when all the data become available after the end of the year. CDC publishes finalized data, such as that above, only after all states and territories have certified their reports. Finalized data for a given year are generally not available until the fall of the following year.

[MMWR=Morbidity and Mortality Weekly Report. The true number of cases of Lyme are underreported, as many are misdiagnosed as having other diseases. The number of new Lyme cases per year is estimated to be ten times that which is actually reported.]

What is a surveillance case definition?

Reporting of all nationally notifiable diseases, including Lyme disease, is based on standard surveillance case definitions developed by the Council of State and Territorial Epidemiologists (CSTE) and CDC. The usefulness of public health surveillance data depends on its uniformity, simplicity, and **timeliness**. **Surveillance case definitions establish uniform criteria for disease reporting and should not be used as the sole criteria for establishing clinical diagnoses, determining the standard of care necessary for a particular patient, setting guidelines for quality assurance, or providing standards for reimbursement.**

[Emphasis was added by the author. Timeliness? What happens to cases that are not submitted "timely"? Note the poignant statement "Surveillance case definitions...should not be used as the sole criteria for establishing clinical diagnoses, determining the standard of care necessary for a particular patient, setting guidelines for quality assurance or providing standards for reimbursement."

And yet that is EXACTLY what is happening in the Lyme arena. Physicians follow CDC guidelines to diagnose; Insurance companies are limiting or denying treatment for Lyme based upon these criteria. Disabilities are denied due to the lack of ability to validate the disease, and Medical boards are prosecuting physicians for treating Lyme patients longer than 30 days because of misinterpreting these guidelines.]

Listed below is the National Surveillance Case Definition for Lyme disease as listed by the CDC in 2006:

[3]Lyme Disease (Borrelia burgdorferi) 1996 Case Definition

Clinical description:

A systemic, tickborne disease with protean manifestations, including dermatologic, rheumatologic, neurologic, and cardiac abnormalities. The best clinical marker for the disease is the initial skin lesion (i.e., erythema migrans [EM]) that occurs in 60%-80% of patients.

[in truth it is less than 40%, and varies in presentation]

Laboratory criteria for diagnosis:

• Isolation of Borrelia burgdorferi from a clinical specimen or
• Demonstration of diagnostic immunoglobulin M or immunoglobulin G antibodies to B. burgdorferi in serum or cerebrospinal fluid (CSF). A two-test approach using a sensitive enzyme immunoassay or immunofluorescence antibody followed by Western blot is recommended.

[Bb is not easily isolated, is not always present in spinal fluid or blood, and testing is not yet reliably accurate, so many Lyme patients fall through the cracks.]

Case classification

Confirmed: a) a case with EM or b) a case with at least one late manifestation (as defined below) that is laboratory confirmed.

[Most doctors do not recognize Lyme symptoms or rashes, and labs do not have the ability to confirm many manifestations, whether early or late.]

Comment

This surveillance case definition was developed for national reporting of Lyme disease; **it is not intended to be used in clinical diagnosis**.

[The CDC makes this statement very clear, emphasis added]

Definition of terms used in the clinical description and case definition:

• Erythema migrans. For purposes of surveillance, EM is defined as a skin lesion that typically begins as a red macule or papule and expands over a period of days to weeks to form a large round lesion, often with partial central clearing. A single primary lesion must reach greater than or equal to 5 cm in size*. Secondary lesions also may occur. Annular erythematous lesions occurring within several hours of a tick bite represent hypersensitivity reactions and do not qualify as EM. For most patients, the expanding EM lesion is accompanied by other acute symptoms, particularly fatigue, fever, headache, mildly stiff neck, arthralgia, or myalgia. These symptoms are typically intermittent. The diagnosis of EM must be made by a physician. Laboratory confirmation is recommended for persons with no known exposure.

[Why 5 cm? So a rash smaller than 5 cm does not fit the criteria? Why limit it to that size?]*

• Late manifestations. Late manifestations include any of the following when an alternate explanation is not found:

• Musculoskeletal system. Recurrent, brief attacks (weeks or months) of objective joint swelling in one or a few joints, sometimes followed by chronic arthritis in one or a few joints. Manifestations not considered as criteria for diagnosis include chronic progressive arthritis not preceded by brief attacks and chronic symmetrical polyarthritis. Additionally, arthralgia, myalgia, or fibromyalgia syndromes alone are not criteria for musculoskeletal involvement.

• Nervous System. Any of the following, alone or in combination: lymphocytic meningitis; cranial neuritis, particularly facial palsy (may be bilateral); radiculoneuropathy; or, rarely, encephalomyelitis. Encephalomyelitis must be confirmed by demonstration of antibody production against B. burgdorferi in the CSF, evidenced by a higher titer of antibody in CSF than in serum. Headache, fatigue, paresthesia, or mildly stiff neck alone are not criteria for neurologic involvement.

• Cardiovascular system. Acute onset of high-grade (2nd-degree or 3rd-degree) atrioventricular conduction defects that resolve in days to weeks and are sometimes associated with myocarditis. Palpitations, bradycardia, bundle branch block, or myocarditis alone are not criteria for cardiovascular involvement.

• Exposure. Exposure is defined as having been (less than or equal to 30 days before onset of EM) in wooded, brushy, or grassy areas (i.e., potential tick habitats) in a county in which Lyme disease is endemic. A history of tick bite is not required.

• Disease endemic to county. A county in which Lyme disease is endemic is one in which at least two confirmed cases have been previously acquired or in which established populations of a known tick vector are infected with B. burgdorferi.

[The author finds the definition of terms used in the CDC's clinical description and case definition, problematic. After reading them, I am left with many questions. Why is laboratory confirmation relied upon so heavily by physicians, when laboratory testing is still unreliably accurate? Why does the CDC stop short of alerting physicians to the problems of accurate testing and interpretation when many doctors rely upon test results as a diagnostic tool? Why is the validity of the symptoms of Lyme, (i.e. encephalomyelitis) being weighed so heavily against the results of testing that is known to be problematic? For example, Bb and antibodies of same are not always present in the CSF or in serum. What

happens to those cases? What happens to Lyme patients with cardio involvement who only present with one cardio manifestation? The definition suggests those patients are ruled out for Lyme with cardio involvement. Indeed, a number of symptoms above are direct manifestations of Lyme, but do not occur simultaneously, and vary greatly between patients. The presence of any of these combination of symptoms should be a helpful clue for the physician to consider Lyme disease. Physicians are often, (my case is a good example), unaware that Lyme is endemic in their area.]

What are the Symptoms of Lyme Disease?

These are the most commonly reported symptoms of Lyme disease, (in layman's terms), and are quite a bit more than what the CDC and other agencies define as criteria for Lyme.[4]

- Known exposure to a tick bite
- Circular rash at bite site that spreads outward or rashes in other parts of body, not necessarily ring-shaped; raised rash
- Sore throat and/or flu-like symptoms, especially in the summer; swollen glands
- Mild or severe headaches or migraines; pressure in sinuses or head
- Unexplained hair loss; scalp painful to touch; feeling of "hair hurting"
- Twitching of facial muscles or other muscles; facial paralysis or Bell's palsy symptoms; tingling of facial muscles or nose
- Pain in jaw/stiffness; pain in ear or neck; stiff neck; tooth pain
- Pain or swelling in or around the eyes; sensitivity to light; double or blurry vision; flashing lights or spots in visual field
- Diminished hearing in one or both ears; ringing/buzzing sounds; hypersensitivity to sound
- Joint pain or swelling; stiffness in muscles or joints; bone pain; muscle cramps

- Irritable digestive system; diarrhea, nausea, pain, constipation
- Pain in the chest, back, ribs; shortness of breath; heart block or arrythmia; palpitations, extra or missed beats; or panic attacks
- Night sweats; unexplained fevers (high or low) or chills
- Shaking, tremors, vibrating feeling or feeling jittery
- Burning, stabbing or biting pains in any part of the body
- Weakness, fainting; or balance and coordination problems
- Partial or complete paralysis, one or both sides of body or in extremities; loss of speech ability or motor skills
- Poor balance, dizziness and problems walking
- Numbness in body; tingling sensations or pinprick feelings
- Lightheadedness, woozy feeling or increased motion sickness
- Hypersensitivity to movement; loss of awareness of body in time or space
- Mood swings, irritability, sudden outbursts, or rage
- Unusual or sudden depression, irritability, suicidal/homicidal thoughts or nightmares; paranoia
- Incontinence issues; loss of bladder function or control with multiple trips to the bathroom at night
- Visual hallucinations; seeing people or things that are not really there
- Disorientation and memory problems; feeling or getting lost
- Feeling like you are losing your mind; scattered thinking, loss of ability to concentrate or focus
- Confusion; problems with communication, or processing thoughts
- Slurred or slow speech; stammering; dyslexic speech or writing
- Going to the wrong place; forgetting how to perform simple tasks you would otherwise know how to do
- Loss of interest in sex; sexual dysfunction
- (Females) Unexplained menstrual pain, irregularity; unexplained breast pain or discharge

- (Males) Testicular or pelvic pain
- Unexplained weight gain or loss; change in ability to eat; sudden allergies to foods, chemicals and other substances
- Extreme fatigue; changes in overall body temperature (too high or too low)
- A flu that you had but after which you never feel well again
- Your pain migrates (moves) to different parts of your body
- Inability to fall or stay asleep or excessive sleep; day-time sleepiness

The MMWR (Morbidity and Mortality Weekly Report) stated:
[5]In 2001, a total of 17,029 cases of LD were reported to CDC by 43 states and the District of Columbia... In 2002, the number of reported cases increased 40% to 23,763 cases... All states except Hawaii, Montana, and Oklahoma reported cases during 2002.

Twelve states reported an incidence of Lyme disease that was higher than the national average in both 2001 and 2002: Connecticut, Delaware, Maine, Maryland, Massachusetts, Minnesota, New Hampshire, New Jersey, New York, Pennsylvania, Rhode Island, and Wisconsin. These 12 states account for 95% of cases reported nationally.

[The reality of Lyme is that its underreported. It is estimated there are approximately ten times the number of new Lyme victims annually than are reported to the CDC. If there are 20,000 reported annually, then 200,000 new Lyme victims appear annually. 200,000 is the entire 2005 estimated population of Walworth County, WI (where the author was infected with Lyme), plus all of Dodge County, WI (where she currently resides.[6]]

The February 11, 2005 issue of MMWR states the following:
[7]**Notice to Readers: Caution Regarding Testing for Lyme Disease**
CDC and the Food and Drug Administration (FDA) have become

aware of commercial laboratories that conduct testing for Lyme disease by using assays whose accuracy and clinical usefulness have not been adequately established. These tests include urine antigen tests, immunofluorescent staining for cell wall-deficient forms of Borrelia burgdorferi, and lymphocyte transformation tests. In addition, some laboratories perform polymerase chain reaction tests for B. burgdorferi DNA on inappropriate specimens such as blood and urine or interpret Western blots using criteria that have not been validated and published in peer-reviewed scientific literature. These **inadequately validated tests and criteria** also are being used to evaluate patients in Canada and Europe, according to reports from the National Microbiology Laboratory, Public Health Agency of Canada; the British Columbia Centres for Disease Control, Canada; the German National Reference Center for Borreliae; and the Health Protection Agency Lyme Borreliosis Unit of the United Kingdom.

[To me this sounds like a little bit of panic on the part of the CDC and FDA–what are they afraid of? Is their concern stemming from the possibility that they are uninvolved in those processes and therefore cannot control their use? What is the motivating factor here, is it patient safety or profit; that is my question...]

In the United States, FDA has cleared 70 serologic assays to aid in the diagnosis of Lyme disease. Recommendations for the use and interpretation of serologic tests have been published previously. Initial testing should use an enzyme immunoassay (EIA) or immunofluorescent assay (IFA); specimens yielding positive or equivocal results should be tested further by using a standardized Western immunoblot assay. Specimens negative by a sensitive EIA or IFA do not need further testing. Similar assays and recommendations are used in Canada. In the European Union, a minimum standard for commercial diagnostic kits is provided by

Conformité Europeéne (CE) marking; application and interpretation guidelines appropriate for Europe have been published.

Health-care providers are reminded that a diagnosis of Lyme disease should be made after evaluation of a patient's clinical presentation and risk for exposure to infected ticks, and, if indicated, after the use of validated laboratory tests. Patients are encouraged to ask their physicians whether their testing for Lyme disease was performed using validated methods and whether results were interpreted using appropriate guidelines.

[Emphasis added. Bolded paragraph is valid. However physicians do not assume Lyme disease, but hesitate to diagnose and treat Lyme, favoring other diseases instead. They say the patient's illness is "all in their head." The fear of the consequences for treating Lyme disease prevent proper diagnosis and treatment. In any regard, the patient suffers needlessly due to the shortsighted and narrowly defined criteria.]

This information is reported on *Emedicine's* web site in 2006:
[8]Lyme Disease Frequency:
• In the US: Lyme disease is most frequently reported in northeastern (Massachusetts to Maryland), midwestern (Minnesota and Wisconsin), and western (Oregon and California) states.

[Lyme has been reported in 49 of 50 United States and also in Canada and other countries.]

(Emedicine continues)... The true incidence of Lyme disease remains vague, as overreporting due to the nonspecific clinical presentation. Lyme disease is increasingly reported because of enhanced physician awareness and sophisticated laboratory surveillance...

[Is the true incidence of Lyme vague because of "overreporting" or is it increasing because of "sophisticated laboratory surveillance"? If there truly is enhanced physician

11

awareness and such surveillance, why can't Lyme patients find any doctors to treat them? This article was contributed to by a Professor at the Medical College of Wisconsin. The article goes on to say...]

Mortality/Morbidity:

• Approximately 80% of untreated or inadequately treated patients develop some manifestation of disseminated disease. Although such episodes are typically subacute and transient, infrequent cases of chronic, severe, and disabling disease have been described.

[From where was this information garnered? If it is known that untreated patients are disseminated at such a high rate, why are doctors so hesitant to treat it? Why is Lyme such a bad word? The article continues on to reveal more...]

• Although 15-55% of patients with Lyme disease report chronic or intermittent symptoms persisting for months to years after **adequate antimicrobial treatment**, recent data do not support postulations of a poorly defined post-Lyme syndrome...

[Emphasis added by author. "adequate antimicrobial treatment?" There is currently no way to quantify what constitutes adequate treatment, Here is my personal favorite statement from this article:]

• Death is rarely, if ever, attributed to Lyme disease.

[Really, there are many families out there who would vehemently disagree with this statement. The CDC reported only six [9] deaths attributable to Lyme disease for the U.S. in 2002, but at least they reported those 6. The numbers are much greater annually.

And last but not least, this statement from the Wisconsin Department of Health's web site:]

[10] Does past infection with Lyme disease make a person immune?

Past infection does provide some immunity, but that protection is relatively short-lived...

[Boy, I must have missed something there, forgive me but I cannot resist. Perhaps the half-life of the "protection" incurred is .0000000001 seconds, and therefore barely detectable. I am not an expert, but I am willing to bet that our damaged immune systems provide virtually no immunity; and with multiple exposures, the disease state worsens exponentially...just ask Lyme sufferers who have been bitten multiple times.]

And what do we do as Lyme patients when the Infectious Disease Society of America (IDSA) has diagnostic guidelines that won't even acknowledge that chronic Lyme exists? "The consensus of the Infectious Disease Society of America (IDSA) expert-panel members is that there is insufficient evidence to regard 'chronic Lyme disease' as a separate diagnostic entity."[11]

As a Lyme victim, I feel compelled to state the following: with all of the misinformation, suppression of facts, denial and disagreement appearing throughout the internet and within the medical community regarding Lyme disease, it is no surprise to me that Lyme patients as well as their doctors are misled and confused about this illness.

Why might I ask, aren't more dollars being spent toward research and treatment into this very serious, very epidemic disease? Why are little-known and/or rarer illnesses that do not affect nearly as many people, receiving the bulk of attention and funding? Is it because our livestock, for example, which are so seriously affected by illnesses such as the West Nile virus, are more "precious" a commodity than we human beings?

Why are Lyme patients being ignored by their doctors and told that Lyme is "nothing to worry about" while these victims suffer needlessly for years and then end up on long-term disability, costing billions of dollars, or worse, dead? These questions are my personal conjecture, but are nevertheless valid.

There seems to be so much information available about Lyme disease, and yet there appears to be no cohesive agreement about how to diagnose, treat, and cure its patients. As a result, patients, on average, wait 2 to 4 years and have to visit up to 20 doctors before their Lyme disease is finally diagnosed. Many of them cannot get proper treatment because of financial and/or insurance problems. Many become disabled, or unable to lead productive lives if they can actually work at all.

For myself, it took 12-1/2 years just to *obtain* a diagnosis for myself and my 2 children. I visited close to 100 different doctors and even the Mayo clinic in Rochester, MN. None of them diagnosed my Lyme, despite my repeated insistence for years that I was exposed to a tick; and my long clinical history of Lyme symptoms.

By the time I was finally diagnosed, I was partially paralyzed on my left side, had permanent nerve damage to my face and hearing in my left ear, and suffered nearly all of the symptoms of disseminated Lyme. When I finally received IV treatments for my illness I could not walk across my living room without complete exhaustion. I know many of you have been where I have been, or worse.

I did not qualify for disability until I had a diagnosis of Lyme disease, and had to quit working for a full year and a half before benefits were finally allowed. Once I obtained a diagnosis, disability only considered all the *misdiagnoses* I had been given previously, as a cause for my disability. Social Security refused to include Lyme as a "valid" diagnosis in order for me to obtain benefits. My disability representative actually stated, "its not important whether you have a Lyme diagnosis or not. I need to determine if you are disabled." To him I replied that it actually *was* important that I had a Lyme diagnosis, because that was the illness that was *making* me disabled!

So before I was diagnosed with Lyme, I did not qualify for benefits, even with all the misdiagnoses that were actually my Lyme symptoms. As soon as I received a diagnosis of Lyme however, suddenly I could qualify for benefits but–just as long as Lyme disease wasn't included in the mix. That did not make, and still does not make any sense to me at all. Why is Lyme disease such a dirty word to disability?

Subsequently I was penalized for a full year's worth of benefits for whatever reason I am still unclear, but it had something to do with my inability to prove that I was disabled for the first year and a half, (meaning no diagnosis of Lyme)!

I admit there are many unanswered questions that arise concerning Lyme disease and it will take some time to sort out the mess that has become the current diagnostic and treatment protocols, and insurance and disability criteria for this disease. But until the community-at-large becomes united in its approach to diagnose and treat this illness, the patients will remain lost in the controversy and political quagmire that Lyme disease is at present.

I submit to everyone reading this book that the state of affairs regarding the diagnosis and treatment of Lyme disease is a disgrace and completely unacceptable in this modern age of medicine. And I ask that everyone join together to enact legislation at the federal level to protect physicians who diagnose and treat Lyme victims. We must end the discrimination of Lyme patients and their doctors, on *all levels.*

We are not cattle. We are worth more than cattle. Lyme is not "all in our heads". We are *real* people struggling with a *real* disease. In case you do not believe this fact, please visit the web site, www.LymeLeague.com. It is an on-line repository for Lyme patients from the United States and Canada, where we honestly tell our very complex, very personal stories about Lyme and our struggles to obtain a diagnosis and treatment.

And a word to those who feel that Lyme patients can be swept under the rug, it is far more *cost-effective*, not to mention compassionate, to heal us than to ignore us.

In case nothing phases you from this book, then I volunteer to donate some of my blood and/or tissue for your own personal use the next time you require a transfusion or transplant. Then you too, can know first-hand what chronic Lyme sufferers go through. You'll learn that not only does it exist, but just how debilitating it truly is. Then we'll see just how far *you* get with 30 days treatment of oral antibiotics, or your insurance company, or your disability office...**Do I have your attention yet?** ❖

Chapter 2

The Forgotten

The poem or should I say prose rather, (that follows in this chapter) was written by me at 2 o'clock a.m. recently when sleep seemed a hopeless impossibility.

The thoughts and emotions expressed within it are echoed by nearly every Lyme patient at some point during their disease process. The author has sadly experienced every single aspect of this work except for one that she was fortunate enough never to have experienced, (being found wandering, speaking unintelligibly and then being hospitalized). But had she not received the intravenous antibiotics when she had received them, she may have quickly added that experience to her list as her own. Make that two. I don't have a service dog, but my great dane, one of three dogs, does provide much needed support and I do lean on her from time-to-time, if that counts. But for those who *have* experienced this illness, the poem provides them with a voice. It reaches out to those with Lyme disease like a hand through the darkness and pulls them back into reality. You are *seen*, you are *valued,* and there *is hope.*

The poem, over the course of just a few days, made its way around the Lyme community and was permitted to be reprinted in several books and publications, distributed to support groups and shared among Lyme patients all over the United States and Canada.

It even made its humble presence known to several Congress members as they met with Lyme support group leaders to discuss cosponsoring Lyme bills already in the House and Senate. Wisconsin is just 1 state out of 49, not currently having laws to protect Lyme doctors and their patients. Currently only 1 state has that distinction, Rhode Island. Two other states, California and

New York were able to have some policy language added to their current legislation, but there are no laws to protect patients nor their doctors for diagnosing and treating Lyme disease. Not even in Connecticut, where Lyme disease was first diagnosed and from where (Lyme, CT) the disease got its name.

I am honored that the work was as well-received as it was intended to be; and hopefully clearly unmasks the face of Lyme for those who do not understand or perhaps do not wish to see.❖

The Forgotten

I am not crazy
This is not all in my head
I am not making any of this up
I am not a hypochondriac
I do not seek attention or fame
I do not have borderline personality disorder
I don't need a psychiatrist or a psychologist
Why do you admonish me when it is you who does not understand?
None of this is my fault
How can you say that my disease does not exist?
Why do you say it is not in my town?
Hush, keep it down or panic will ensue
People might move away
Or worse yet, never come and visit
We can't have that can we?
I stand here before you as a testament to my illness
I am a helpless victim of a cruel disease
And an even crueler system
Your misdiagnosis is designed to render a pill so I go away
You choose to ignore me and I will go away
Eventually I will die of a disease called ignorance
If the illness doesn't get me first
Some die by their own hand out of desperation

Many have tragically lost hope
You see the dark circles under my eyes and say that I must be tired
You have no idea of my tiredness
Not half as tired as I am of hearing that I don't exist
That I am invisible
Or that I am nuts
Or that I do not matter
You say you don't believe in my disease
But it believes in me
Let's take stock of all that my imaginary illness has given me
The gift of my experiences and the toll they have taken
I am allergic to most foods, and many medications but not really,
My body just thinks it is
I am not a basket-case, but I do feel like one
I have seen 10 doctors, or 20 or 50 or 100
None will give credence to me
I have every illness known to man except that which I truly have
According to them
I don't smile because my face has nerve damage
You interpret it as looking mean instead
I try to communicate but it is work for me
You think I have an attitude problem
I can eat only five foods for months at a time, or four,
Or sometimes only one, but this isn't a diet
You don't understand
And you make me feel bad about my food "choices"
I run screaming out of the store because the light bothers me
There is terrible bone pain
I can no longer use my limbs
I have no sex life
I suffer panic attacks and palpitations
I have a heart block or arrythmia or chest pain
Fatigue so profound I feel like the walking dead

Hello you say on the phone in my moment of silence
Did I hear what you just said? I can't as I'm quietly seizing
Blanking out, a moment of ceased function
You hardly notice, you think me not listening
I wear sunglasses in the daytime not to be fashionable
I can't stand sound at any volume or I cannot hear at all
Motion sickness plagues me, my stomach my enemy
Turn me in circles and I get confused, disoriented, dizzy
I struggle to regain my physical strength
Desperate for human connectedness
A kind word, an understanding heart
Save me from this isolation I feel
An unwelcome blanket of silent uncertainty
You say I am wanting attention
Tumors appear in me for no apparent reason
My organs are failing while you call my blood work "normal"
My ears ring incessantly; my eyes no longer work
Or I can no longer see
My head hurts worse than any migraine I have ever had
Even my hair hurts
I wince when you touch me, when you kiss me
I need reassurance but your embrace is painful to me
Or I find none at all, feeling your rejection from lack of support
Because I am too much work
Because you are tired
Or you have had a long day
You walk out on me
I have no value to you
Because you do not comprehend
Strange sensations, odd tastes, odd smells that are not really there
I have lost my hair and not from bad hair genes
Lost weight, wasting away because nourishment escapes me
I feel biting, stabbing and jabbing pain in my body
Nails of fire are burning my skin, a red-hot poker
I feel bugs crawling on and under my skin

They bite me relentlessly but I cannot see them
Excuse me while I die, one cell at a time
I am being eaten alive, from the inside out
My immune system is thwarted by something I cannot control
My brain manipulated, my body stressed
This thing controls every aspect of me
I see the world through a filter
My thoughts are dark, sometimes suicidal, you call me insane
And then elation, roller-coaster mood swings which have no meaning
I am so cold, hypothermic,
Or feverish, wet from night sweats or chills
My joints and muscles hurt, ache, throb, burn, and are swollen
Who are these people I am hallucinating? I know they do not exist
Yet I see them before me, standing there, threatening me
I am paralyzed, I am incontinent,
I am a shell of the person I used to be
I can't breathe, or eat, and I can't think straight
Words fly out of my mouth that I did not choose
I am dyslexic, I am speech-impaired, I cannot speak at all
I forget where I am going, what I am doing, and who I am
I am confused and frightened
I lose my temper from nothing at all,
And I fight with everyone for reasons I can't explain
The night hours are long and I cannot sleep,
Or I sleep longer than I should
I fall asleep in the daytime and need to rest throughout the day
I stumble along falling, knocking things over
You tell me to be careful
I have no perception of myself in time and space
I cannot control my own movements
I am called disabled by some; others refuse to label me that
You accuse me of crimes I have not committed
Like failure to work
Failure to pay child support
Failure to show up places

Argumentativeness
Impatience
Like it is really a choice I would make
You reject me because I am unreliable
Because you don't understand
I am sorry I missed your family function
Or party, or funeral, I was too sick to attend
You say I am not sick and my disease is but my imagination
I have rashes on my body that are hideous and uncomfortable
I cannot eat; my toilet is a valued friend
I am hyperactive, or a slug, laying about each day
I have trouble learning new things
Or remembering them
When you poke me with a needle, my blood won't flow
I am so tired of the tests, the needles and the drugs
The home remedies, the sure-fire cures
And emptiness of the unknown
I am spastic, I twitch, I jerk, I tremble, I shake
I can't lift a milk carton, or dress myself, or comb my hair
My teeth hurt and my gums and nose bleeds
I have bruises all over my body and I don't even know why
When I look in the mirror, I no longer recognize the image there
The person I was is now a shell of my former self
I have lost my children, friends and family
Because they just don't understand
Maybe I can no longer work, uncertain how I will survive
I've lost my livelihood, my home, my finances, my health,
And my future
I cannot get disability because my illness is not on the list
Or maybe I have disability but it still doesn't help pay the bills
I have filed bankruptcy or live on the verge of it
I cannot get insurance because I am ill but no one will say that I am
I cannot go to doctors because they don't want me there
Or I have the wrong insurance
Or worse yet, none at all

Family courts have punished me
Taking away my children
They tell me I am playing games
Because I cannot work
Because I endlessly reschedule hearings
Because I struggle with my memory on the stand
You accuse me of heinous crimes
And take advantage of me
To get what you want, my children
Because you can and they let you
Because I am ill
Maybe you found me wandering in the street
Speaking insanity, out of my mind
You accused me and put me away
Shame on you
Yes I am still sick
Is this taking too long for you? I am sorry
I don't know if I can be cured
No there are no tests to see if I am well
I cannot find a doctor to treat me
Or diagnose me
Or care
This never should have happened
It could have been avoided
If you had just listened to me
And tried harder to help
I can no longer drive, walk, think, write or function,
Or enjoy any part of life
I have a service dog
Or maybe I can't afford one
I can't stand up or walk straight
I am depressed
I am lost in a sea of despair because no one sees me
I am invisible though I stand before you.
You close doors in my face and send me away

Because you don't want to deal with me
Because you say three weeks is enough and I should be cured
Or worse yet you experiment on me without knowing what or why
Because you are afraid of being a doctor
Of losing your license to practice
Hesitant to being compassionate
Or afraid to pass a Bill
To take governmental control
To assist your constituents
Because no one wants responsibility
To be forced to acknowledge that I am ill
Like it is some sort of a crime
I did not choose this disease
It chose me (oh lucky me)
To you I don't look sick, but I assure you that I am
Outside I look fine, but inside I am screaming
I am angry
I have a right to be
Let me explain
I am the forgotten
I have Lyme

by PJ Langhoff   ❖

❖ Chapter 3 ❖

Introduction

I spend the majority of my nights writing. That is what I do at two o'clock in the morning, when I cannot sleep. It happens to me an awful lot and I usually spend approximately the battery life of one portable laptop computer's power typing away. That comes to about 4 hours 3 minutes and 42 seconds, or two good evenings of really creative writing if you don't count the time it takes to demolish a bowl of plain popcorn and pick the crumbs off of the bedspread. I have to get everything important off my chest as quickly as possible before the fatal "beep" noise warns me of the battery's impending shutdown.

Secondary to that process, if I don't write down my thoughts, they become lost to the wind, or to the moment, or all time. Then I become destined to spend the remainder of the evening or morning hours, solving my problems while in delta wave state.

Let me make myself clear – just because I think my thoughts, does not make them important or great. But rather, the thought alone of the formation of those ideas is what is so important to me. It is exactly what I can create with these random ideas that seduces me into recording them for later use.

The activity of thinking is actually a wondrously phenomenal process that should be fully exploited by everyone. It is a useful creative process to be examined and protected, molded and savored. I personally don't want to waste a moment thinking random thoughts without jotting them down so that I can perhaps use them in some manner on a future date, hopefully for someone's greater good.

This commentary is not a morbidly delusional, self-induced hypnosis that has me believing I can save the world or that my words are vitally profound to the betterment of mankind. I am not recording my most intimate mental creations just because I am at the top of the hill in age and descending downwards as some testament to my life or the need to leave behind some narcissistic legacy.

I am certain that my high school creative writing teacher, whose name I have sadly long since forgotten (sorry), or her quasi-prophetic statement that I would be a "really great writer some day" still provokes me like some guilty phantom from my past to whom I must forever answer.

But I do believe that our thoughts, even random ones in the wee hours of the morning, are a little piece of our spiritual essence. They are a spark of our divine self that we cast outward like stones upon the water. And like ripples in a pond, our thoughts affect every aspect of whomever they touch and wherever they are cast.

As such, thoughts are extremely powerful things. Negative and positive thoughts alike can, and have ruled worlds, ruined nations, brought peoples of all races together, or segregated and destroyed millions with their toxic hatred.

All the greatest things in life that have ever been created, (at least by mankind), have all begun their either meager or fantastic existence with a simple random thought that somebody quite simply, thought.

So getting back to thinking and writing, my ranting along in these pages here actually began its life as me complaining on paper or on the screen at least, about most of the symptoms that I had experienced due to Lyme disease.

But then my personal thoughts-are-things mantra kicked in and I realized that my words were far too negative. So I went back and changed them into something with a distinctive direction. This was a conscious choice on my part, and why the heck not? I could take these words and either wastefully complain away the day and they would become useless, perpetual residents on my hard drive, or I could weave them into something useful; breathing life into my creation to the point where someone might actually want to read what I had to say.

In some small way, I hoped that my words might resonate with a fellow Lyme patient who was perhaps feeling lonely, or depressed, or even invisible (there is a terrible lack of understanding toward Lyme patients and the effects of this disease on them.)

And then something happened. I sent the words to my poem out in the morning's email message to my support group members who also have Lyme disease. I hoped that maybe I'd hear a "gee that sounds like me", or an "oh gosh, I'm glad you put a label on such-and-such for me".

What I found instead was an overwhelmingly positive response spreading throughout the Lyme community like a California wildfire, and all from a seemingly innocently inspired work of 2 a.m.-ness on my tiny little laptop computer.

What I saw manifesting before me were the very real results of my rant-turned-positive-thinking decision randomly and purposefully affecting the lives of Lyme patients all across the United States. How way-cool was that? One person can indeed make a difference. I inherently know that anyway, but here was proof-positive that positive thinking could spark a reaction in others. *(And take that mom, you always said no one wanted to hear what I had to say!)*

So the next time you are feeling small or unseen, speak up. Remember we are each powerful beings and we have the right and responsibility to make this world a better place to live in. Each voice is important, each person critical to building a "kinder, gentler nation", one person at a time.

I always thought when I reached over-the-hill status, that the achievement was something of which to be proud, an accomplishment of great esteem. By then I should be married, have three children, a station wagon, a dog, a large house in the country, a healthy savings account and a hefty portfolio.

Well, I had 2 horses, 3 dogs, a cat, a rabbit, 4 birds, 3 fish and a chicken. I had a portfolio but it was empty and dusty and laying on top of the file cabinet. I had just filed bankruptcy for the second time in my life, published my second book that nobody knew about yet, and ran a couple of support groups for Lyme patients. I had a dollar and thirty-three cents in my purse, a headache, and nobody to take out the garbage for me.

Our house was in the country (sort of); well, a really small village nestled in the heart of farm country, about 18 miles from any major town in any direction. Not quite what I dreamed of when I was a teenager, but as things go, not the worst of places I could be in my life, either.

I also had a diagnosis of Lyme disease, never what I imagined to have when I turned 45, and facing what I considered to be the second-half of what was supposed to be the *easy* part of my life.

In truth I was married, (for the second time), I had two children who no longer lived with me, an ex-husband in league with the devil, his bull-dog attorney dumpster-diving in my supposedly private medical records in a misguided attempt to prove me mentally ill and an upcoming appointment with a forensic psychologist to prove in court for the fourth time (ad nauseum) that I have no, and was never diagnosed with, mental illness of any kind, and especially not that which was now alleged to be as "caused" by Lyme disease.

Yes, Lyme disease and the ignorance and discrimination surrounding it can make you crazy, but not the kind of crazy that they were accusing me of. I had no mental illness from Lyme disease nor anything else. There was not even a history of mental illness in my family, not that it is anything to be ashamed of, illness is illness.

But the family court system in beaucolic Walworth County, Wisconsin was allowing these two men to manipulate the court system in order to discredit me by whatever means they could fabricate, including publicly scrutinizing my medical records in order to do so.

Gosh, now you too can look up my records and see just how many warts I have had removed from my left foot (3). Or witness for yourself the results of my recent pap test (negative). Let's send out a press release about that and see how many really want to know, shall we?

My favorite pieces of information that are now a permanent part of public record (and I voluntarily share them with you here to show what **lunacy** is allowed for discussion during trials in the family court system), are the accusations my ex-husband made of me that included these tidbits: that my decision to have breast implants years ago was somehow a lifestyle choice that now makes me ineffective in my role as a parent. This statement was objected to in court, but instead of being rapidly assuaged, the comment was instead, glorified with a five minute on-the-record discussion validating those concerns.

Or better yet, this one: his claim that I have a large tattoo of a tongue on my crotch actually became part of our trial testimony as well. The judge allowed it despite our objections, but I ask you again, what does that have to do with my parenting role?

Actually I *do* have a tattoo, but it is on my lower left hip. What it is, is really nobody's business but for those of you who don't have the time to peruse my very public life thanks to more than a decade in the Wisconsin court system (and still counting); it is similar to the Rolling Stones' famous lips-teeth-tongue logo, though a tad modified so as not to infringe upon any copyrights.

So I have implants and a tattoo, so what. That doesn't make me less intelligent, more radical, mentally ill, or incapable as a parent; nor define my value system, my intelligence, nor my character. So I have a nicer looking rack after donating the top half of my figure to my two lovingly breastfed children. And I have a tiny quarter-sized permanent reminder of quiet rebellion on my left hip, big deal. Then of course there is the plain truth that I have a diagnosis of Lyme disease (and co-infections), which should be just about as inconsequential within the family court system as the other two very personal items are, but sadly is not. At any rate, any of the above information has *no business* being exposed in family court by a misguided, angry man and his wayward attorney.

Neither should I have to repeatedly submit to the humiliation of being tested numerous times for a supposed mental illness all because my ex makes unfounded accusations due to my Lyme disease. Indeed, when I have already proven three other times that I have no mental illness I have to return to court to do the same thing for a *fourth* time. But the court foolishly allows his behavior to continue unrestrained, costing tens of thousands of dollars in attorney's fees in order to defend myself.

I should also not be required to sit and listen to a judge say that I am in contempt because I cannot remember the right things to say when I am testifying on the stand. The fact that I have Lyme disease and cannot answer questions properly depending upon the degree of my brain fog on that particular day should *never* lead a judge to admonish me for being "evasive", or allow him to accuse me of playing "games".

As the so-called privacy laws currently stand, any yahoo with a penchant for destruction and a desire to be obnoxious can get your medical records and put them on public display, and in this case, be used for personal gain. All that is required is a court-order and a semi-valid sounding excuse.

Any court that would allow an attorney and his (or her) client to claim mental illness against their ex-spouse in an effort to retain custody of children, all because that person has a diagnosis of Lyme disease, or any disease for that matter, is tragic and abusive; and should be punishable and prohibited by law.

The laws simply *must* change when a Lyme patient who, because at the time lacks a diagnosis, is required to sit upon a witness stand, and listen to an uninformed judge state the following: that because I don't have a diagnosis and because I don't *look sick;* because I don't yet qualify for disability, therefore I must not in fact, *be sick;* so "logically" the aforementioned party should *be able* to seek work and therefore the Lyme patient is in *contempt of court* for not seeking work, or for not working.

This is discrimination, ignorance (meaning not knowing), **and a disgrace.** This is unfortunate but represents the system that is currently in place. And that rubs me more than a little bit, in the wrong manner.

Despite everything I have done and been dealt in life, in the time it has taken me to reach the top of that proverbial chronological "hill" and begin my transition downward, I have found more of myself through the process of getting there, and have retrieved parts of myself that were lost to the wrong teachings of my childhood than I had ever thought possible.

For what its worth, due to many of my experiences, I have also cast away the strict religious dogma my upbringing force-fed me and gained a new perspective on life in general, trading a true spiritualism for commercial religion and consumerism for understanding and compassion.

I realized also somewhere along the way, just how integral the events in our lives truly are. Nothing happens by chance and everything contains meaning and a lesson for our spiritual growth. It is only how we choose to interpret the meaning of the events in our lives that provides either a fruitful or a stagnant outcome for us.

For those of you who do not agree with me, just humor me please while you read this book and then see where you stand afterward. You can most certainly disagree with me, that is the beauty of life. We all have options, and choices.

In fact, there is a choice you can consciously make, every day of your life. If you walk around with your eyes shut, you won't see anything but darkness. If you have them open however, you can see your dreams and the dreams of others, manifesting into reality.

I am inviting you to walk with me in *my* reality for a little while to explore the life that I have created through right and wrong choices, "blood, sweat, and tears", joy and pain, accidents and planned events, and of course, being exposed to Lyme disease.

Call it fate, karma, God's will, or whatever you wish, the path that has become my life is one that, although complex and difficult, is one I am personally glad to finally recognize as having been a blessing to me.

Yes, Lyme disease in one aspect, has been a blessing of the greatest kind, for me personally and also, it is my hope, for the many others out there struggling with this very real, very devastating disease. I hope that the issues with which we struggle that I choose to share here in a positive manner, will manifest in a similar fashion as did the poetry written earlier in this book. Hopefully my writing will touch the lives of others in a manner that will raise awareness for the greater good of all.

Bless you on your journey, let's walk together for a while, shall we? ❖

❖ Chapter 4 ❖

The Start of Something Greater

As I sat in the shade of our back yard in Elkhorn, Wisconsin in the summer of 1992, I squinted my eyes and tilted my head upwards toward the bright afternoon sky. The rays were somewhat shielded by the two hundred-year-old oak tree under which I sat, while I supervised my two youngsters playing in their sandbox. My quiet, self-amusing daughter was just three, and she was joined by my thirteen-month-old son, who was actively attempting to load sand into a bucket with his bright orange plastic shovel.

What a wonderful day I thought to myself, as I closed my eyes and felt the mild breeze blowing upon my face. The previous winter, we had moved the entire family up to southern Wisconsin from Chicago, Illinois, after our second child was born.

I had been working full-time third shift while my husband worked seven days a week, days. He really did not have to do that, but he was a workaholic. I kept my job after the children were born because we needed the money, but I was dead tired of working the late night shift and then sleeping an hour or two until my husband went off to his day job. Then I would be up with the children all day long and repeat this schedule over and over. After three and a half years, I was a walking zombie and I was unable to do it any longer.

So when my husband got a job offer to come up to Wisconsin, we took the chance for a better way of life despite my having to turn my back on my good paying job and my husband taking a hefty salary cut. The idea was that I could now stay home and raise the children, and go back to college to finally get my college degree, something that had been elusively dodging me for years.

All my life, circumstances kept getting in the way. First my parents wouldn't pay for my college when I graduated high school. They told me "girls don't need college" while my three brothers were given a better opportunity. Okay, one brother graduated, one dropped out and the other one went into the Army, but I was never given the opportunity in the first place. The truth is that I wasn't given any credence because I was female. Those were the times and that is how it was.

As I grew older and independent, my work hours were not conducive to much schooling, though I would fit whatever classes I could into my already overbooked schedule. Over time, I attempted to whittle down what seemed like an insurmountable amount of credit hours in order to meet graduation requirements.

Later on I got married, and approximately ten months to the day, my first child was born. Even she took the opportunity when she saw it, for I had planned to go to school *before* I had children, but as life would have it, she wouldn't wait. Time went along and parental responsibilities overtook me and I was very happy with that change, though exhausted. My second child, a boy, came along a respectable two-and-a-half years later.

When our infant son was just nine months old, my husband received a job offer in the adjoining state of Wisconsin. The pay was substantially less than what he was currently earning, but enough to support us. With our combined incomes, anyone would have thought us fools to take such a huge pay cut, but we did it anyway. We might have to struggle for a couple of years, but we could manage this new lifestyle if we were frugal. If the choice had been left solely up to me, I would have jumped at the chance to get out of the city.

We had previously tried to make my life easier by hiring babysitters to come into our home and sit with our children in the morning hours so that I could get a few hours of precious rest. In a house barely 700 square feet in size, that was a difficult thing to achieve, but I was willing to try anything.

By the time my husband's job offer came about, I had seen my share of errant in-home care providers and I didn't want to go through that situation any longer, as it had disastrous results.

On her very first day, one female candidate stole my wedding ring. I had her arrested, but sadly not before she had hawked the jewelry at a nearby pawn shop. Another girl stole food, and another one diapers and formula for her granddaughter. One woman acted as if she was planning on kidnapping my child and said many very strange things. She talked about a "bed partner" as she called him, who had supposedly tried to commit suicide the week before, and who was now an inpatient in the hospital's psychiatric ward. The sitter was supposedly visiting him each day after completing her duties with my child. She also incessantly repeated her opinion of how much she *loved* my daughter, how *cute* she was and how much she'd *love to have a child just like her*.

Something in her demeanor felt insincere to me, so believe it or not I actually called the hospital to corroborate her story. I asked if there was a psychologist having the name our sitter had provided. I inquired after the patient she had described as well as the visitation hours she had suggested.

I was told that the information I had been given was false, *all of it*, and furthermore, the procedures the girl had described, were not those adhered to by the hospital, either.

The administrative nurse of the psychiatric unit and I discussed the sitter at length, and collectively agreed that my employee's behavior was not only strange, bit possibly even dangerous to have around; so my husband and I fired her. She then tried to reapply to the very same job she had lost, when we placed an ad for her replacement. She used a false name this time, but I thought I recognized her voice on the answering machine message.

She left a different phone number than the one she had previously used. Somehow I managed to get the phone company to verify who owned her new phone number. After describing with full conviction about my previous experiences and my concerns about this gal, the phone company employee broke the rules. He was able to verify that the number she gave me was indeed her own, and listed under her legal name, and not the alias she had just provided. This woman really *was* trouble with a capital T, and we had been wise to let her go. The lesson here was to always trust my gut feelings.

Another woman we hired, invited her family over and talked on our phone all morning long, while I was in the bedroom attempting to sleep and my children were left unattended. That situation clearly didn't work out and I fired her within the week, but she stalked me for about a month. Courtesy of my mail slot, every few days, I received strange cards containing threats written in crayon. I would also receive phone calls from diet centers or nursing homes saying that I had missed my appointments with them–appointments that I had not made but apparently our ex-sitter had, in order to harrass me.

In hindsight, I think that these persons each represented a test of my patience and understanding, and ability to "let go" of issues that were not important, like the harrassment blatantly flung upon me. I was to learn to hold steadfast to my convictions, trust my gut feelings, and brush off harsh criticisms of ignorance and prejudice. The events also taught me the importance of keeping a close watch on my surroundings and reorganizing my priorities like my family and myself, all valuable lessons indeed.

So as you can see, I would have jumped at the chance to get the heck out of our town (and situation) and get some decent rest, and away from all of the craziness. But I still had to convince my husband that the impending move was something that we *should* do, though I really did not know just how different our lives would be after that decision was made. My hubby considered the job offer for a couple of days and seemed to drag his feet over it. Eventually however, I convinced him to take the deal and I set about reorganizing and relocating our lives.

The move felt strangely natural to me, almost like we were *supposed* to be moving to Wisconsin. I could not explain at the time, why the feeling was so firmly entrenched in my brain that we had to move but I never really questioned it. It *felt* right, like some predestined choice that we were *supposed* to make at that time in our lives.

In what must have been a record setting, two and a half week time period, we had our IL house sold, our belongings packed and moved, and a new home sought, bought and inhabited, and there we were, in sunny southeastern Wisconsin.

Sadly, after less than a year, my husband's new job would fall by the wayside, leaving him unemployed, and our future threatened. In August I un-registered myself from the local college just before the semester began and found myself returning to the workforce in order to support our family. When my husband found a new job, the pay was comparatively smaller, so I had to continue working to keep things afloat.

All in all, life was somewhat better in these new surroundings. I still had a workaholic husband, but at least the children were getting better quality time with their mother. I worked nights now, but only part-time, so I was actually getting some rest while earning a little money. Could things be any better, I thought to myself. Life seemed to be at least a bit more normal now than it had been back in Chicago.

Life was slower here, and more relaxed. I had time to explore with my children. I'd pack them into the car in the morning and we'd set off down the road with a picnic lunch, blanket and my camera. The day was spent exploring and playing in parks or on swings and then we'd return home, with me a little more educated about the area, and with a few new photos and happy memories.

Life seemed pretty good to me at that point, but I really had no idea of the things that were yet to come. Here I sat, nearly a year after we had arrived in Wisconsin, with things a little different than we had planned, but overall, good. There I sat, underneath the majestic 200-year-old oak tree, and peering up at the sun.

My attentions skyward were interrupted by the sudden shrieking of my eldest child, whose face was on the receiving end of a shovel full of wet sand. It wasn't her fault that my toddler couldn't control his arm movements and I quickly instructed her to close her eyes and keep them closed. I quickly told my son that his sister was okay, since his face was now wrinkled in an expression of both fear and concern at his sister's predicament. I really did not feel the need to have to handle *two* crying children.

Hoisting my son onto my hip with one hand and grabbing my daughter's arm in the other hand, I helped them both into the house and dealt with the sand removal process as carefully as possible.

I have to admit that my daughter was very good about the procedure, perhaps because I had remained calm throughout the situation. At any rate, copious amounts of sand were carefully removed from her eyes as I flushed them as gently as possible under the faucet after first carefully dabbing them with wet Q-tips.

"Poor kid, what a rough day you are having. Your brother did not mean it, he can not help what he does, he's just a baby", I told her. A few kisses and sniffles later, everyone was much better.

"What is this on your leg honey?" I would ask my daughter, as I saw what must have been thirty or forty tiny black spots. They resembled some of the sand that had just washed down the drain, so I carefully brushed them off of her calf and went about our day. A few of them were stuck to her skin, but I didn't worry. I figured she was going to have a bath that evening, and I could scrub her legs more thoroughly then.

That evening when it was my son's turn to bathe, I noticed the same dirty dots on his legs. Both children had been wearing shorts that day and both of them had been sitting in the sandbox. Since the sandbox was located underneath the shade of both the oak tree and the tall pine in our backyard, I figured that the specks of black must have been something from one of the trees. I merely scrubbed until they were removed. I had no idea that what I was dislodging from my son's leg, and that which I had removed earlier from my daughter's leg might actually be living, though it was hardly larger than a grain of sand.

A few days later my children both came down with what I thought was a summer cold. Runny noses, fevers, crankiness and the associated symptoms that are common among sick children appeared. I did the usual mom-thing and took the kids to their pediatrician to ensure that their colds were, in fact, merely colds.

The doctor smiled and tried to reassure me that my son's strangely high 106 degree fever was only a manifestation of a virus and prescribed an over-the-counter remedy.

Many days later, my daughter began to complain that her legs itched. Since she was now taking an antibiotic for her supposed summer cold that had lingered more than ten days, I thought that perhaps she was experiencing an allergic reaction to the medicine. At the time, she was taking Bactrim, a sulfa-based antibiotic.

I described her ring-like rashes to the doctor, who confirmed via phone that they were most likely hives caused by the medicine, so we discontinued the treatment. The rashes went away in a few days and her health seemed to improve somewhat.

My son had a similar case of "hives" appear on his legs and stomach. Naturally, the doctor advised me once again, to discontinue the medicine for him as well. "Well, your children *are* related, so they are probably both allergic to sulfa drugs. Is your husband or you allergic to sulfa?" he asked me. I replied that no, neither of us had any allergies. "Well that's it then, he said dismissively. "It must be an allergy of some sort." He ended our visit, and I think if I would have let him, he would have patted me on the head. Was this really an allergy to sulfa? I wondered silently.

Despite the doctor's dismissal of the problem, the mom sentinel inside of me made a mental note of the rashes and filed the images in the dark recesses of my brain. For a while, life returned to some semblance of normalcy.

At the end of that summer, and a few months after the children had manifested rashes on their limbs, I was getting ready for bed. I noticed that I had a tiny black scab on the upper left part of my back, nearly in between my shoulder blades, but more on the left side.

I picked and picked at what I thought was the scab until finally it dislodged and bled a little. Since the removal of it didn't hurt, I thought nothing more of its presence.

But a couple of days later, I experienced what were probably the worst flu-like symptoms I ever had.

I walked around the house nauseated for days at a time. My joints and muscles ached terribly. I was having trouble seeing, thinking straight, and suffering from terrible headaches. I had excrutiating pain in my upper right abdomen and I was running a fever of 104. In the morning I would be drenched, wet from the night sweats I was experiencing. I was also so exhausted that I had to stay in bed for most of the day, leaving the children to run around the house half-dressed, which to them, was wonderful. To me however, it was the hellish beginning of years of illness that would redirect the very course of my life.

Of course I went to my family doctor, right after I drove myself to the emergency room for dehydration and my 104 fevers. The ER did not know what to do and labeled my illness a "virus". They advised me to get a flu shot; why to this day, I do not know, but they did give me a prescription for amoxicillin for a ten-day stint, which I took.

I went next to my general practitioner, because after two weeks, I had developed a large, ring-type rash about the size of a deck of cards, above the part of my back where I had removed the so-called scab. With each day that passed, the rash grew progressively larger until it disappeared from view entirely, absorbed into my skin. But at the first sign of the rash, I made an appointment with my doctor about it.

Due to my children's many rashes, I had done some research in the library about them. In those days there was not really an internet as we know it today, so the only information I found was from the encyclopedia volumes there. I asked my doctor point-blank if he thought that my rash could be caused by Lyme disease. He answered "no", and with that one word, my future would be permanently altered.

I asked him next to hypothesize what *could* be causing the round rash with the big blank spot in the middle. I knew nothing at all about Lyme, but I did somehow recognize the bulls-eye rash that was appearing on my shoulder blade. He said simply, "I don't know, but its not Lyme. We don't have Lyme here in Wisconsin." Little did I know that the doctor's lack of knowledge was going to sling a death blow to my health. He ordered a sigmoidoscopy and a stool culture for me to do, instead of diagnosing or treating me for Lyme disease. He failed to recognize the clinical symptoms of Lyme; you know, the illness that was not *in* Wisconsin, according to him.

After a few days the bulls-eye rash expanded in diameter. I decided to make an appointment with a dermatologist. Perhaps he would know what he was looking at, I reasoned. I was wrong. To make matters worse, I had to wait two full weeks to see him. And in the time it took to get to the day of the appointment, my bulls-eye rash disappeared and would be replaced by a series of smaller, football-shaped rashes, each about the size of a quarter. These new lesions were intensely itchy and would progress from a few on my shoulder, to many covering my entire back, neck and trunk of my body.

The dermatologist concurred with the first doctor that my rash was not Lyme-related, but he also did not know what was causing it. I carefully described the preceding bulls-eye rash that had manifested, along with my physical symptoms. "Probably some form of dermatitis", he would say to me, completely unaffected by my strange illness. He handed me a bottle of a pink liquid, probably calamine lotion that was repackaged so that he could charge me a premium price. "Put this on the rash and it should disappear in a couple of days."

I followed his directions, though I was displeased that two out of two doctors had no idea what was making my skin look so ravaged. I still had an undignified sigmoidoscopy to undertake for whatever reason, I did not know. I was already routinely scraping fecal matter onto a little cardboard collector kit in order to complete the parasitic screen the first doctor had ordered. None of it made any sense to me. It was not my stomach that was causing my skin rashes, why wasn't anyone listening to me? I felt really very ill and no one was heeding my cry that perhaps I had Lyme disease.

While I struggled to feel well with doctors who were on a wild goose chase, I had little time to focus on my own health. My children were busy being toddlers. If my now eighteen-month-old son wasn't happily locking mommy out of the house when I got the mail, he was smearing liver sausage on the white vertical blinds in the living room. This was no time for me to be sick—I had two small children demanding my undivided attention.

My husband finally lost his job, and sat around the house complaining about not finding a job or criticizing the fact that I did not have the laundry finished, or the supper cooked. He knew that I didn't feel well, but lacked required general observational skills and understanding. He never seemed to notice or care, not even when I was in bed for several days at a time.

Sure he'd poke his head in the bedroom and say, "its 8 o'clock, should I feed the kids?" But this was the same man who insisted on stealing my bed in the labor and delivery room because his back "hurt", relegating me to sleep on the room's sofa despite my 9 lb. baby trying to make its debut into the world. (Yeah, the nurses practically killed him for that, and in retrospect, I probably should have let them.)

More time passed with me not feeling my best, even after repeated courses of various antibiotics. But I did achieve a relative wellness where I managed to function, despite my swollen glands and persistent health problems. I still suffered from devastating headaches and odd episodes of intense pain in my upper right abdomen, as well as my joints. I also had difficult menstrual cycles, which had plagued me before I had children, presenting as endometriosis. But the condition had improved since I had delivered my children, though now it seemed to suddenly return, and in full-force.

Despite walking well at nine months of age, my infant son began to stumble and fall much more often than I thought he should. He had also begun to talk but it became apparent from his speech that he was having trouble hearing what he was saying. Sometimes when I talked to him, I could tell that he couldn't hear me, so I thought I'd better get his hearing checked. Remember my husband? He made a comment one day about our son's hearing problems and to this day takes sole credit for saving our son's hearing, and to hear him tell it, his life. If anyone deserves credit to me, it would be the surgeon, or perhaps God Almighty.

An examination at the pediatrician's office confirmed that my little guy's ears were filled with fluid that was not draining. He suffered many nights of extremely high fevers, convulsions, and months of antibiotics before I grew tired of asking the doctor if there was anything else we could do.

I could not justify submitting my infant to permanent antibiotics, so I searched for other options. I finally located a reputable Illinois otolaryngologist (ear-throat doc) who examined him. The doctor indicated to me that ear tubes were absolutely necessary to drain the fluid to the eustachian tubes or else my son could suffer permanent problems with his hearing.

A flat tympanogram confirmed the diagnosis–his hearing was already adversely affected. Three thousand dollars and a set of teflon ear tubes were inserted, the money in the surgeon's pocket and the tubes into my son's head.

The tubes worked for a time, but they kept falling out as he grew. (My son had a second set at age 3 and a third set at age 6. We finally abandoned the process when they fell out the third time.) The first set however, temporarily seemed to quell the walking and communication problems. In retrospect, my own experiences with Lyme-induced vertigo, coordination and speech problems would convince me years later, that my son's symptoms were more closely related to his Lyme disease than anything else. I now wonder just how much the ear tubes masked his symptoms, rather than treating them, and I question whether three surgeries were ever really necessary.

Ear tubes aside, next it was my daughter's turn to exhibit new symptoms when she turned six. Kindergarten was already stressful enough for her, because she was the youngest in her class. She had missed the deadline for entry by only three weeks, darned September birthdays. She was more than ready to attend school; and I knew that. At four she already could write the alphabet, spell larger words, count well and had a sizeable vocabulary.

I had spent a good deal of time with her, sounding out words and teaching her to read and write and she was ready. I wanted to wait to have her enter school because of the possibility she might fall behind emotionally due to her age. In the long run I knew it would be better for her academically if she entered sooner. She was tested by the school and easily accepted for early admittance.

Now the girl who had potty-trained herself at age two, was suddenly having incontinence issues. It seemed that her bladder would deceive her and she started having accidents in school. We worked hard to determine what was causing her problems but never found a medical solution. The doctor said there was "nothing wrong" with her bladder.

He diagnosed instead, emotional problems, citing her early school term as the causative factor. I disagreed with him, for I knew that she loved school. Dissatisfied with his diagnosis but out of options, I hoped the problem would resolve on its own and it did, ceasing just as suddenly as it had started. Many years later I would personally learn about incontinence issues surrounding the Lyme spirochete's attacks upon the bladder and urinary system.

My daughter's problems abated, my son began having the same problem while on medication for his supposed ear infections. Despite his ear tubes, he began to have high fevers again, combined with sore throats, cryptic and swollen tonsils, respiratory infections and skin rashes. Roseola, Scarlet Fever, and even possible Measles were the diagnoses, despite his being properly immunized.

When his fevers arose, I would bathe him in cool water, usually during the middle of the night and I would do whatever was humanly possible to keep him stable and myself sane while he began to experience mild seizures. Antibiotics and then stronger antibiotics were prescribed. No testing of any kind was done, no diagnosis rendered, no guess ventured. Everything he experienced was blamed on that darned ear fluid, though in my gut, I felt it to be something more.

After the doctor had suggested that my son's incontinence was caused by his current medication, another doctor told me that his incontenance was *not* a side-effect of that medication, so naturally I was confused. I had no idea what was going on with my son medically, and I couldn't understand why the doctors couldn't at least agree on the cause of his bladder dysfunction.

Time has a way of fast-forwarding into the future if we don't watch what we are doing. Although the children's bouts with fevers, upper respiratory infections, rashes, bladder dysfunction, nightmares, sleep disturbances, and anger problems arose and continued, they seemed to disappear into the background as my own health continued to disintegrate.

The year was now 1994, a full two years after we were infected with Lyme. I had been to several more doctors, endured yet more tests, and spent a couple thousand dollars to boot. Most exams focused on my gastrointestinal system since I was having great difficulty with that. Because of my abdominal pain, I also had scans for my gallbladder in case there were stones, but none were ever found. Despite that, my side continued to erupt in terribly debiliating pain approximately every 3-4 weeks and I'd spend days holed up on the couch or in bed with heating pads welded to my stomach.

I had been to the hospital emergency room a few times already because of not being "well", and was treated for dehydration. They told me to drink more water after providing me with rehydrating IV fluids. Sometimes I would receive a shot in the back side and a prescription for one antibiotic or another.

At this time high fevers began to reappear. I would awaken in the night, wet with sweat. And, quite frankly, I can say that during a few of these episodes, there appeared to be *people* walking around in my bedroom, which I found unbelievably disturbing. These random nighttime hallucinations were frightening and for the first time in my life I thought maybe I was going nuts. Back to several more doctors I went, but none of them would venture a guess as to why I was having nighttime visitors. The general concensus was simply that I was under too much stress.

I do admit there was an awful lot going on in my house. When my husband had lost his job, he sat around with few hopes for new job prospects. We lived in a small town and he was twenty years my senior, and at the age of 53, he was not an easy-sell in a new career field.

We had taken our meager savings account and combined it with a bank loan and a few credit cards when my company laid me off, and I purchased computer equipment to start my own desktop publishing company. To jump-start my business, many of the clients that my former employer had enjoyed were left stranded when the business went under. This allowed me to contact them and pick up where my ex-employer had left off. I had an instant home-based business; and it was very successful due to a ton of hard work on my part.

I worked long hours at the keyboard, but managed to do it around my youngest child's naptimes, and transporting my oldest child to half-day kindergarten five days a week.

To make matters more complicated, after my father had passed away, my mother sold our family home in Illinois and decided she would move up to Wisconsin to be near her only daughter, me. I did not want the arrangement very much but my husband insisted that she and I could work out our differences and have a happy relationship, albeit late in life.

My mother had done the best she could I suppose, but there was a long history of abuse in our family and though I tried to bury those demons in the past, mother seemed to tenaciously cling to the idea that I was perpetually twelve years old and that she had never done anything wrong in her life, including being abusive. Her twisted perceptions made her believe that I was not living my life up to her standards and she carefully reminded me of that fact almost daily.

Despite my insistence to my husband that mother wouldn't last a week in Wisconsin, he pressured me into convincing her that it was a good move. Overruled, I honestly gave it everything I had, and hoped to turn over a new leaf with her. It was my sincerest wish that we could find some common ground. Although I honestly knew that it probably would not happen, I was mature enough to be willing to try.

I helped her to pack her things, sell her home of twenty-six years, and move into a house just across the street from us and down two homes. She was within walking distance to the town, doctors, dentist, and us. Despite this, mom insisted on having me drive her everywhere.

Her idea I suppose was that since she was retired and had some money to spend, that we would rekindle our relationship (if we ever had one at all) by going shopping, her favorite past-time.

What really happened however, was that I became her chauffeur and had to submit to her demands and her whim. I felt responsible for having brought her to live near us and she exploited those feelings whenever it suited her. It increasingly seemed like my family, and especially the children's needs, were to take a back seat to mother's whims of antique hunting or grocery shopping. Of course I did not agree with her position on that.

I visited mother every day and included her in every activity, though she rarely wanted to partake, choosing instead to spend her time alone indoors with her elderly dog. She appeared on our doorstep exactly three times in the entire five months that she lived in Wisconsin before she decided that she was unhappy living here and wanting to return home to her friends in Illinois.

Because my health was such a mess at the time, and because my husband was largely responsible for urging her to move up near us, I left it up to him this time to pack her things and move her back down to Illinois. I had had enough of her inconsiderate demands, and I was through with trying to please her. I had enough to worry about with the two children, a fledgling business and a physical state that was rapidly going down the toilet.

I think what made matters worse for mom was the fact that I had recently admonished her for forcing me to take her home first before I stopped in to retrieve my son from kindergarten, which made me five minutes late and my son very upset. He thought his mom had forgotten him, God bless his little heart. No, it wasn't my memory that was at fault, not yet. It was his grandmother not wanting to sit in the car for a couple of minutes so that I could pick him up on time. Her butt was apparently more important than my son's feelings and shame on me for putting her selfishness first at the time, I am sorry my son.

In the end, my husband saw my mother off to Illinois while I, from her perspective, ignored her completely. She didn't make any effort to call her own daughter or stop in to say goodbye, either; so she was as much at fault as was I. Meanwhile I was forced back into bed, and suffering from undiagnosed Lyme disease.

Yes, there was an incredible amount of stress in my life at that point, but I didn't agree with the doctor that my hallucinations could have been caused purely by stress. I had suffered many things in my earlier life which had included unhealthy doses of stress, and I had always handled those events as best I could, and that manner didn't include fabricating imaginary people walking about my bedroom.

I continued searching for another doctor who might actually listen to my complaints and concerns that I possibly had been exposed to Lyme disease. I found a rheumatologist in nearby Burlington. Although she agreed with me that my symptom history could indeed be Lyme-related, she hesitated to do any testing or prescribe antibiotics because of all the previous ones I had taken. She told me they should have been enough to "cure" Lyme, if indeed I had ever had it in the first place.

I visited still more doctors. I was successful in convincing a doctor in 1995 that he should at least "pretend" that I had Lyme and treat me as if I did have it. Although he also would not test me, he prescribed a combination of amoxicillin and tetracycline, which I took concurrently for over a month.

I did reach another plateau of comparative wellness, but then I intermittently began to have problems with what resembled panic attacks. Suddenly out of the blue and often while driving, I would begin to experience a rapid heart beat. I would feel flushed and warm, and sometimes I would even seem to have trouble breathing as well. The episodes were terrifying, especially when I was out driving on the highway with my young children in tow and no one around to help me. Cell phones were still a luxury item then and I did not own one yet.

I had several of those episodes that year, but none of the physicians to whom I described them, could identify their cause. My EKG's were always normal, and so was all of my blood work. Stress was blamed for a lot of my symptom history, and many doctors tried to tell me I was quite simply, depressed. Despite my telling one doctor that I did not feel the least bit depressed, just very busy and very ill, he prescribed anti-depressants anyway. I ripped up the prescription as I angrily left his office.

I was learning that whenever doctors could not determine the answer to a woman's illness, they often immediately assumed she was delusional or depressed and therefore, in need of medication. I absolutely hated the medical profession back then and my general feelings about doctors haven't changed much since that time, although I was happy to learn that there are many excellent doctors out there; I just had not run into any of them yet.

After a few years, I lost track of the number of doctor visits I had, and the many tests I endured. I could rattle off medical terminology like it was nobody's business from all of my research and personal experiences. I even managed to take a course in medical terminology at the local college so that I could more easily understand the words and their meanings that I was reading. However, I still did not know very much about Lyme disease, because there didn't seem to be much information out there about it. Besides, every doctor whom I had asked, had insisted that I couldn't possibly have it.   ❖

❖ Chapter 5 ❖

Away We Go

In 1997, shortly after my mother returned to Illinois and we moved to our second home in Wisconsin, my then-husband decided that he no longer wanted to be married and walked out. There were other circumstances surrounding that event and many unfounded accusations on his part, but the fact remained the same. I was left with a huge mortgage and no viable means of support. Months earlier, I had been forced to close my business upon my husband's insistence that I spend more time with the family, and because my health was continuing to spiral downward, I had agreed. I see now that it was his way of really sticking it to me, as I learned later on that he had been planning on leaving even before we purchased the new home.

There I sat in a huge house on five acres of land in the middle of nowhere, with two small children, ages six and nine, and wondering just where we were going with the rest of our lives.

Adding insult to injury, my soon to be ex-husband was playing many games within the court system, like hiding income, selling off marital assets to friends and then later retrieving them; stalking me incessantly and causing property damage; hounding my friends with questions about my whereabouts and just plain being a major pain in the you-know-what.

As routine family court matters would go, both my spouse and myself were to submit to court-appointed psychological examinations in order to determine who was best suited as the custodial parent. In short, my psychiatric profile noted that I was under stress due to my husband's harrassment of me, but that I was perfectly sane and fully capable of objectively and properly raising my children. My husband on the other hand, did not receive as favorable a review, I am sad to report. Although I cannot disclose the contents of the actual report, I *can* tell you that it was deemed an "invalid clinical profile", repleat with apparent lies designed to make himself look good to the examiner.

There were notations about his recent behaviors including the forcible removal of my children from a day care provider while not his allotted visitation time period along with other dalliances and poor choices on his part.

The long and short of our custodial arrangements were that we were awarded joint custody with me as the parent with physical placement and him as the parent with a liberal visitation schedule and child support obligations.

This judgment did not sit very well with my ex-husband, (especially the monetary part), so he vowed verbally that he would "make my life worse than a living hell" and he began to do anything and everything in his power in order to exact that threat.

He continued to stalk me for years, and yelled loud obscene comments at me in public when picking up or dropping off our children. During my son's first communion, my ex shouted vulgar obscenities at me while in the church vestibule, for no apparent reason other than the fact that I had the audacity to ask him what time he was planning on returning our children after his visitation had ended.

During Mass, my ex was videotaped sitting one row behind us, muttering unkind things about me under his breath. He also set about squashing my son and I in the aisle on the way to communion to the point where I directed our son to walk ahead of his parents due to his father's obnoxious behavior.

A scene caused by my ex at the children's school picnic was another experience that required the principal to call the police. I wasn't even present at the time it occurred in case you think I had anything to do with it.

My ex had a penchant for dissension and an anger management problem, and my children and I were thrown into the middle of it whenever he saw fit. My ex loved to play games designed to create a negative paper trail about me, and to my dismay, there was very little I could do to stop him.

Over time, the police even took to driving by my house and blinking their headlights as a nod to let me know that they were around. My ex had forcibly entered our home long after he had moved out and frightened the children and threatened a friend of mine.

Although I requested the police to issue restraining orders against him, my request was not granted because he wasn't "doing anything" harmful that could actually be proven. I guess entering my home though uninvited, causing flat tires the night before every court hearing and property damage that appeared out of nowhere was considered acceptable by the police.

Sadly, my mother and brothers began to side with my ex because of his artful skill at fabricating lies. I did not spend very much time arguing or defending myself with them, because he had already convinced them I was the guilty party. Slowly my family began alienating itself from me; at least until years later when half of them finally saw my ex for the person that he is. In the meantime, I was very much alone, and unsupported through what I then thought was the toughest part of my life. In truth, it was just the beginning of a very long journey for us all; physically, emotionally and spiritually.

This is not an attempt to berate my ex-husband (although he probably deserves it), for what he has done in the past and continues to do in the present, it is merely setting the stage to illustrate the kind of behavior that is tolerated from a certain male parent who finds himself under the jurisdiction of the Walworth county family court system.

None of my ex's behaviors, although proven by witnesses many times, ever elicited the least bit of admonishment from judges or family court commissioners. Even when he was proven to be lying in court, the judges turned a blind eye to his antics, and allowed him to pursue his claims against me, no matter how ridiculous or unfounded those claims might be.

Among other things, I remember when he lied about receiving money from my grandmother to help him pay off some bills, when the poor woman had already been dead for more than two years–and during the time the loan was supposedly rendered. Doesn't the word perjury come to mind?

As a parent, and especially as any good parent would feel, one of the most outrageous things you can hear about yourself in court are false accusations that you would "kill" your own children if they were left in your care. Most people would find a statement like that utterly ridiculous, coming out of the mouth of an attorney as directed by his client. However, a court commissioner, at one point during our pre-trial, actually took those words very seriously, despite my having no prior criminal history nor would I ever for that matter, (that claim left open to interpretation as you will find later on in this book).

I included this information not to be sardonic, but so that in time, you will see that I have never been granted the same consideration that my ex has been given in the family court system. These happenstances are essential in order to illustrate the incredible discrimination that abounds within the courts. It exists not only against female parties to an action, but more specifically, *ill* female parties to an action, and struggling with an illness as complex and controversial as Lyme disease.

Our divorce was finalized in 1998 and I would have placement of the children for five full years before the original custody and placement arrangements would be turned completely upside-down.

After some time, I found a temporary job working for a publishing company located in northern Illinois, about 60 miles south of my home. Since I lived only about 4 miles north of the border of IL and WI, I accepted my only job offer.

Because of the recent move to our new home before the

divorce, and the traumatic disappearance of their father from their lives only weeks after our move, I felt it imperative that the children retain some continuity somewhere in their lives. Despite the distance and inconvenience, I made the decision to keep them in the same school they had attended the previous year until I figured out where we would live permanently.

Every morning, we would get up early enough to eat breakfast, and get ready for school. I would drive the children 18 miles to their old school, drop them off, and backtrack to the highway near our home, and continue east to a doggie day-care center where I would drop off our adopted greyhound. I felt eleven hours in a kennel in the basement of our home not entirely suitable for the fellow. I decided to choose daycare for him instead, considering his feelings as part of the family. After that delivery, I would venture south into Illinois through heavy traffic, often speeding in order to get to my job on time.

Somehow for months I managed to spend eight relatively productive hours working per day, then I repeated the morning run in reverse at quitting time. Most days were a mad rush to get back to Wisconsin before the daycare center closed at 6:00 pm, but I always managed to get there.

To this day, I don't know how I coped with the 176 mile round trip every day, as my Lyme symptoms were manifesting in new and unusual ways. I was having trouble concentrating, and my panic attacks while driving were becoming unbearable. Still, you do what you must when you have to do so, and I plodded along often sweating and white-knuckled from fear, as best as I possibly could.

Eventually, I would have to surrender our marital home due to pending foreclosure, but that was fine with me because I could perhaps find a job closer to home and we could move somewhere less expensive that had real people around us, and where I could still work but not be forced to commute so far.

As it would happen, upon discovering my financial situation, my creative ex-husband who previously had reported to the courts that he had no money whatsoever; entered a motion to retrieve our marital home, to rescue it from foreclosure. The court allowed him to take it away from me with no questions asked, while leaving this mother and her two small children without a place to live.

My ex apparently *did* have enough money to pay the fourteen hundred dollar a month mortgage while I did not. Oddly, the court never questioned him about the discrepancy over his previously reported paltry income and his statement that he made in the beginning of our divorce that he could not afford to live there (no doubt to dodge alimony and child support).

Suddenly he was fully capable of paying not only the reduced child support he managed to have ordered, but also the $1400 a month mortgage, the $5,000 septic system lien and the $6,000 in back house payments to bring it out of foreclosure—and nobody noticed that except for me.

As you probably suspected, once he moved back into the home, I automatically lost any equity I might have been awarded and the marital property he supposedly had sold to his friends mysteriously reappeared in the driveway (a corvette, a couple of motorcycles and a train collection included as part of the booty).

My ex was living like a fat cat in a huge house on several acres of land with multiple vehicles in his possession. He paid a paltry sum of child support based upon his underreported income, and he got away with this behavior for years.

Meanwhile we had to make due with no income, living off the remainder of my surrendered IRA, what little I had left after being forced to use it to make the house payments over the previous year. Jobless, I now sat facing bankruptcy, in debt to my eyeballs. There were back business bills and taxes from a partnership my ex was never held accountable for. There I sat with a mysterious illness, two children and no place to live, and that was just fine by the family court system and everyone in it.

I managed to work an offer in compromise with the federal government for the now $15,000 in back taxes after truthfully explaining our divorce situation and the fact that I had virtually no money. With debts finally satisfied, I concentrated on my children's welfare and how to deal with my ex's shenanigans every weekend when he would visit our children. I did eventually find employment.

From 1998 until the spring of 2000, I dated several people, though I was not interested in any permanent relationship. But my best friend who lived next door to me in our newly rented Milwaukee home, persisted in convincing me to go out on a date with a good friend of hers. Although he was a nice man, I quickly decided that he was way too quiet and besides, he dressed funny, so I wrote him off as a future dating prospect.

Over time however, the powers that be presided and managed to persuade me to take a second look at him. He was always around, which I found out later was by design, and he was helpful with handyman work around the house whenever I needed it. He was also a mechanic, and it was a relief to have someone to work on my car when it needed it. Due to my ex-husband's frequent tamperings, it broke down regularly and my budget did not allow for extra car repairs. But I was so badly damaged emotionally from my marriage to my ex that I did not have another marriage in the forefront of my mind.

I had endured years of abusive behavior from the man who had fathered my children, including one episode of rape that his attorney stated in court had "never happened," just because I hadn't bothered to call the police at the time it had occurred. The court agreed. There had been no police report, therefore it must have never happened, and I was accused of lying about the incident when my accusations finally surfaced in court, years later.

When he raped me, I had just had breast implant surgery and was still in bandages and unable to lift my arms above my head. Despite this, my husband clearly and forcibly attacked me despite my obvious wishes otherwise. During the process I could barely struggle due to my surgery, so he easily pinned me down with his arms, although I repeatedly yelled "no" and was utterly terrified of him. The angry and dominating expression of contempt on his face clearly indicated that I had no choice in the matter and I felt absolutely violated, not to mention that I was in pain.

The process actually ripped two stitches out of my surgical area which led to me losing a little blood. The pressure upon my chest made the previous medical insult to my body much more severe than normally expected from the process. When my surgeon had mentioned something during my later follow-up appointment about my extensive bruising, I declined to explain why that was and let him think instead that it was related to the surgery. (I did take photos of my injuries at the time.)

After the rape, I felt horribly dirty, frightened and abused, and I remember crying in the shower as I attempted to wash off the feeling of disgust that I now had painted upon me. Later when I implored my ex to tell me why he had done what he had, he said sarcastically, "because I felt like it."

Because the rape happened just prior to my ex abandoning the family, I was concerned that my young children would have a father in jail. Although I *should* have put the man in jail, I felt at the time it more important that my children's father *not* be in jail, because of the potential emotional harm it could do to them. Had I known his intentions to desert us, I probably would have changed my thinking, because then he would no longer live in the same household. I also did not report him because I was afraid of him and the consequences of doing so once he got out of jail. He was capable of practically anything and I knew it.

During our marriage, this was the same man who had exhibited many angry outbursts and attempts to kick down the locked doors that myself and my children sometimes huddled behind. This was a man who, with me and our small children in the car, would purposely drive on the wrong side of the highway, towards oncoming traffic, in an attempt to prove a point or control me. This man would ram his shopping cart into others at the supermarket because he didn't like the way someone parked their cart in the middle of the aisle and he was not about to wait for them to move it. In our inner world, the man was hostile to me and our children but to the outside world, he was capable of incredible poise, self-control and charm.

In the long run, the decision not to report the rape was not the best I know now, because he was never held accountable for his actions and he absolutely should have been. If I *had* reported the rape, in retrospect, I don't think he would have *ever* been grant-ed placement of our children, under any circumstances. Wrong as it had been, I nevertheless made my choice, and have had to live with the consequences of that decision, ever since.

So here I was, a couple of years post-divorce and although I was getting back on my feet financially, I was still hurting emotionally. The friendship that this new man offered to me was one of a mutual respect, kindness and a sense of peace like I had never known in my first marriage. Eventually the man broke down the barriers that I had against him and we became not just friends, but really good friends. I told him that was all I could give him at the time, but that was good enough for both of us to call it a marriage. We were engaged and married in 2000.

Just before our engagement, I came down with an upper respiratory infection that would not go away. I was having great difficulty breathing and had been on antibiotics for months. My doctor, assuming chronic bronchitis, prescribed an inhaler filled with steroids to help me with my breathing. Unfortunately, this was the wrong medication to give to a Lyme patient, but remem-ber, nobody knew then that I was suffering from Lyme disease.

The inhaler actually caused my breathing problems to grow considerably worse, and I ended up in the hospital where I was treated with yet more steroids and a shot of a penicillin in the hiney.

My fiancé and I tried desperately to discover the source of my respiratory problems. About the same time, my son began experiencing the same sort of symptoms, and he too ended up using a rescue inhaler.

Eventually we located a colony of black mold living under the stairway to the basement and alerted the landlord of the home we were renting. The owner did nothing about the situation, so I was left to bleach the offending areas in order to erradicate what we thought was the cause of our ailments. We did recover somewhat after that, but my airway was left with a permanent wheeze.

In 2000, after returning home from a camping trip, I noticed a red rash on my scalp. A few weeks later and about nine weeks before my second marriage, I began to suffer from pain in my left ear. I went to the doctor who diagnosed me with an ear infection. Over the course of the next five days, my ear pain manifested into a hugely inflamed left ear, with pain that radiated from the top of my head on the left side, all the way down my left arm, shoulder and back, and down to my waist. (In Lyme disease, this is known as Borrelial lymphocytoma.)

If you touched my skin, I would wince in excrutiating pain. Air that passed over my skin's surface was painful to me. There was a persistent fullness in my inner ear, and I was dizzy, making it extremely difficult to walk. Slowly, the feeling in my face went numb and I found myself unable to close my left eye, move my facial muscles or my mouth. In under a week, I became paralyzed on the left and central parts of my face, and I lost my sense of taste and smell to boot. Speech became extraordinarily difficult, I was having trouble swallowing and I suffered excrutiating pain. I had never before seen anything like what I was experiencing. All that the descriptions in the medical books could suggest was Bell's palsy, though the other symptoms I suffered from were distinctly absent from those pages.

I visited five different doctors at the clinic over the course of the next five days and each one had a different diagnosis for me. No one seemed to have a clue what was wrong with me. First they diagnosed an ear infection, then cellulitis of the ear, and finally migraines. Shingles of the cranial nerve without pustules was diagnosed by one physician.

I was prescribed oral steroids and acyclovir. After only three doses, my body went into anaphylactic shock. I thought I was going to die on the way to the hospital. I was having trouble breathing and began to black out. By the time my husband and I stumbled into the ER, my lips were a lovely shade of blue, and numb from hyperventilation.

I was told I was experiencing an allergic reaction to the medication I had taken and was directed to stop taking the drugs and the "problem" would go away. I did, but it didn't.

The new pain in my face and ear was unlike anything I had ever experienced before. I sat at work with a heating pad literally pasted to the side of my face for weeks in order to try to ward off the incredible discomfort. To make matters worse, the look on the faces of my co-workers was so embarrassing to me that I took to covering my face whenever I had to speak or laugh, because I was frightening to look at, especially when I laughed.

My employer didn't seem to understand that I was ill, and scolded me repeatedly for taking so much time off of work. In fact, I had many vacation and sick days coming to me, and I utilized those until they were exhausted. But from the perspective of my employer, I was never around, and that is all he remembered. Eventually, my facial paralysis reversed itself, but in its wake was permanent nerve damage to several parts of my face. It is difficult for me now to smile to any extent and my face has a natural expression of disdain etched upon it, through no fault of my own. Since it is harder for me to use my smile muscles, photographs tend to make me look stern and people see me as angry or sad looking, when I really am not that way at all.

Later on in court, I would be accused by social workers as having "eyes of pain", and several times it was noted that my face had a "flat expression". I was even accused by the social worker of having a face "full of rage". In court, my stern looks were repeatedly blamed as a manifestation of some deep underlying emotional problem needing to be addressed, rather than what was actually true, evidence of Lyme damage to my facial nerves.

People's perception of me because of my facial nerve problems would permanently be altered by Lyme disease. To me it was bad enough how I would find myself treated when in public with a paralyzed face. I would have to endure stares whenever I tried to speak. It was necessary for me to repeat myself when words wouldn't come out clearly and shop keepers would talk to whomever was standing next to me, instead of directly at me when I would ask them a question. They would do this ostensibly pretending not to notice my disability when in reality they were visually put-off by my appearance.

I could not understand why I wasn't being treated in the same manner as a "normal" human being, because I sure felt like one, albeit a very sick one. While I was already compassionate enough as a person to understand ridicule of the handicapped, this one life lesson alone opened my eyes to the disabled person's perspective. It really hurt to be treated as somehow less than "normal" and that lesson will stick with me always.

In the summer of 2001, I was having great difficulty at work due to my Lyme disease flare-ups. I had painful problems on my left side that I thought were left over from my supposed shingles of the cranial nerve. Doctors called it post-herpetic neuralgia, or PHN. All I knew was that I was in agony all day long and my left arm and hand were no longer functioning properly.

I went back to my general practitioner, and asked him to please run some tests to find out why I was in so much pain all the time. He complied and actually ran every kind of test he could possibly think of. He included allergy screenings, heavy metals, nutritional profiles, you name it, I had it done. I even dredged up my history of Lyme-like symptoms and urged him to test me for Lyme disease. His response was that even if I ever was exposed to Lyme disease, I wouldn't have it "now" because I had been on so many different medications over the years that it would be cured. But he ran a Lyme titer anyway. To my dismay, it came back negative, which he interpreted as meaning that I did not have Lyme disease. Unfortunately the doctor couldn't have been more wrong in his interpretation of that test.

There are those that would defend his actions and say that he did enough diagnostic work to rule out Lyme disease. But I submit to you that his findings were not the *benchmark* of whether or not I had Lyme, but instead, *just a test that failed to show Lyme at that moment and that one time alone.*

Seeing someone with a long clinical history of Lyme-like symptoms and especially when a tick bite and rash were noted, should raise a red flag to any doctor about the possibility of Lyme and every avenue should be pursued with that as a possible diagnosis. Because of the seriousness of long-term Lyme disease, the disease should no longer be dismissed on the basis of one or two lab tests alone, tests that are still not yet 100% accurate.

The CDC states that "The diagnosis of Lyme disease is based primarily on clinical findings, and it is often appropriate to treat patients with early disease solely on the basis of objective signs and a known exposure."[12] In my case by the time 2001 rolled around, I was probably well past the throws of an early disease process, but if any one of the previous doctors I had seen had attempted to treat my claims of Lyme exposure with any credence in the beginning when I was exposed to it, I might not be writing this book today.

There were also other tests available in 2001 that might have helped to rule out Lyme disease besides the Lyme Titer. In any case, a multi-tiered approach to testing may have proven fruitful, even several years after my exposure. "Low antibody titers are often perceived by doctors as meaning that their patient is somehow less sick than someone with a high titer. Actually the opposite is true. Someone with a high titer means that they have a greater natural immunity."[13]

So someone with a low or negative titer could just have a high viral load, or else they could not have been exposed to Lyme at all. At any rate, the tests are not 100% accurate, and doctors must be careful when interpreting them. Again, the patients' medical history and history of exposure to Lyme *must* be taken fully into account.

My frustrations with my doctors paled in comparison to the pain that riddled me all day long. I lost sleep at night because I could no longer lay on my stomach or left side. I had to sleep on my back. When I awoke, my left arm or hand or sometimes both hands would be asleep.

I pursued referrals to several neurologists and an osteopath. It was determined that I had pinched nerves so I was ordered to undergo several months of physical therapy in order to alleviate the problem.

When the first round of physical therapy proved more painful than my symptoms, it was ordered that I halt therapy and rest for a few months. After which, I would resume the therapy sessions.

Therapy or what was supposed to be therapy designed to achieve wellness, began to cause other symptoms that were undesirable. The left side of my face began to act strangely, and I was now having spasms of the facial muscles. My eye would twitch uncontrollably as would my shoulder and arm muscles. Eventually the twitching grew painful as my muscles could no longer rest between spasms. This produced terrible muscle tension headaches that lasted for days at a time.

After one court hearing, my attorney noticed my "winking" at him and thought perhaps I was being overly-friendly. During one hearing, the rapid movement of my left shoulder in an up-and-down motion had to be controlled by my other hand, because it was distracting to those on the witness stand. Although I may have appeared to be faking my illness to some present during the trial who made comments to that end, I assure you and them that I was very much in the throws of neurological Lyme disease and the effects it was having upon my very heavily infected nervous system.

I still did the best I could to continue my physical therapy, at least until the point where I was beginning to have terrible pain in the left side of my face. Fearing the worst of my facial paralysis returning, I begged my doctor to remove me from physical therapy and in frustration, he did.

To his knowledge, he had tried everything that he possibly could to diagnose what was causing my pain and health issues, and at this point, my credibility was down the tubes. I began to notice comments within my medical records that said things like "patient is hypersensitive", or that patient "appears depressed", or "difficult". Sometimes the Medical Assistant would pre-screen me and write observations in my chart like the fact that I had my eyes "averted" or was "looking downward" as if it was some technical fault meant to assist the doctor in diagnostics for depression screening (it was).

Solely because the doctor had no answers to my illness, I was indeed diagnosed as depressed and my doctor tried numerous times to tell me that I needed anti-depressants in order to treat (or mask) my symptoms that were in his opinion, basically psychosomatic, or all in my head.

My doctor would not pursue the Lyme diagnosis, and actually had the audacity to say to me, "Look, I'm not going to hold your hand every time you think you have something wrong with you." I was so disgusted with him that I told him what I thought of that remark and walked out of his office that day, in tears. Unfortunately for me, my insurance at work pretty much designated who my primary care physician could be and the clinic was only two blocks from my home. I was now too sick to drive very far so I had to continue to tolerate his verbal abuse and obvious contempt for me as a patient.

Getting back on the subject of employment, work became increasingly more difficult. To make matters worse, I had recently badly sprained my left ankle one night after awakening to a visual hallucination that caused me to rise up and stand on top of my bed. Because I was not yet fully awake, I stepped off the tall king-sized bed in the full darkness and landed on the side of my ankle from a height of nearly three feet. As you can imagine, I heard the crunching sound of injury but that paled in comparison to what I was hallucinating, which sent me running downstairs in a blind panic. It was only after I awoke fully that I found myself in excrutiating pain from my injury. At work I spent six weeks of icy winter, having to negotiate three floors of stairs several times each day while on crutches, despite my inability to hold them properly because of my failing left side.

My boss was finished tolerating my accidents, injuries and illnesses, and he looked for the first opportunity to get rid of me that he could find. Unfortunately, there began almost a conspiracy to get me–me, the manager who had received the highest merit bonus ever at that same company, the previous year. Now the upper management staff was looking for any excuse to get me to leave, including requiring me to work longer hours, refusing me time off for illness, all but literally holding the door open for me to leave.

Their efforts caused an undue amount of stress for me as you can imagine, and as Lyme was rearing its ugly head in full force, the stress added to my symptoms. As a result, I suddenly grew, (and Lyme aggravated), what was now an extremely short fuse.

Out of thin air one morning when I was feeling particularly miserable with Lyme symptoms, another manager said something to me that was entirely inappropriate. I fired back words that I would never have otherwise utilized in what I can only describe as having been caused by the Lyme infecting my brain. In a sudden and inexplicable rage, I told him to go relieve himself of any sexual tension (although I didn't use those precise words), and then I walked out the door.

Before I knew what had happened, I found myself without a job. Curiously, the company was offering to "settle" for a large lump sum for my being *allowed to quit* because they didn't have real grounds to fire me, but they did want me to leave. I told them I wanted to return to my job but they didn't want me there because of my attendance issues. Eventually they renegged on their offer of a settlement, so I filed for unemployment compensation instead of receiving any lump sum.

In a state of confusion about the situation, we did have to go through an unemployment hearing that eventually denied me benefits on the grounds that I had supposedly been "insubordinate" towards the manager, despite the fact that I did not work under, nor report to him and he was considered same-level management.

In the end, the owner of the company who was my boss, decided that I had been taking too much time off of work, and said as much at the hearing, so my job was history. I was left without a job, settlement, or unemployment benefits–and I did not even know how the incident had occurred nor what had set me off in the first place (Lyme rage).

Of course my ex-husband took every opportunity to take advantage of the situation in which I now found myself. I bet you thought he fell off into the background since a few years had passed since the divorce was finalized. No, unfortunately he was just waiting on the sidelines for something to utilize against me; anything, and this was the perfect situation for him to exploit.

My illustrious ex, always searching for new and clever ways to discredit me, must have found out from the children that I was no longer working. Apparently he found the phone number of my ex-employer and had a discussion with him, which blew my socks off when I learned about it from my unemployment attorney.

In the past I had already witnessed my ex checking up on me at work through our business internet sites. Apparently he was unaware that I was the manager in charge of the on-line order department and that I would also see the catalog request forms that he continually submitted in an effort to scope out exactly what it was that my company manufactured.

My attorney informed me that my ex had offered to my employer, the ability to place my young son upon the witness stand in order to help prove that I could not perform my job, and thus bolster my ex-employer's unemployment case against me.

I then learned that my ex had claimed (as if he had some kind of first-hand knowledge), that I had been staying up all night long, and working long hours in my home in order to try to learn new skills I supposedly did not have, but needed in order to do my job properly. If I *had* been doing that, then I say, good for me, but in reality, I was not doing anything of the sort.

Good God, I was the former Director of Internet Operations for a large manufacturer/distributor and not only did I manage a handful of people, but trained thirty-some employees how to effectively utilize our company's eight web sites I had designed and created with my team. I routinely wrote computer code in several languages and designed and implemented interactive software programs for our company.

I was hired from a subcontracting position and asked to head up the internet department and later, the graphics department as well. In addition, I had other skills my ex would only dream of understanding, (the computer-illiterate creep).

And now he was claiming that our ten-year-old son would have some critically supportive first-hand information about my supposed employment shortcomings (that didn't exist), and that somehow my ex-boss *could* or *should* feel free to utilize my son's testimony in order to help prove his case against me and withhold unemployment benefits.

Exactly who was the nut-case now? I wondered. I could not believe my ears when my attorney told me this. She did not know anything about our divorce case at all, so I knew she would have had no motivation whatsoever to invent such an outrageous story.

Who on earth in their right mind would attempt to do such a thing anyway? Had my ex-boss contacted my ex-husband to try to dig up whatever dirt he could on me? For the life of me, I couldn't imagine him doing anything of the sort. Despite his personality shortcomings, my ex-employer was basically a good man.

No, I thought, that was not it. What I could absolutely see happening however, was my ex-husband contacting my employer, in order to attempt to harm me in any way possible.

We did have an upcoming hearing in which my ex would later accuse me of "walking away from a $50,000 a year job", as if it really mattered to him that I had done that.

In reality it did matter to him, because it would seem that he had already been working behind the scenes in order to set the stage for what he would initiate down the road through the court system.

Whatever the arrangement, I was far better off without either one of those men, and facing the stronghold that my Lyme disease was now establishing–and in a manner I could no longer pretend to ignore. ❖

"Do what you feel in your heart to be right,
for you'll be criticized anyway.
You'll be damned if you do
and damned if you don't."

– Eleanor Roosevelt

❖ Chapter 6 ❖

A Bump in the Road

As if the stressful problems with my employment and ex-husband were not enough to keep me busy in life, my Lyme disease began a full frontal attack on my health and well-being in the summer of 2001.

Since I was now without a job, I actually had much more time to spend at home with the children, who were out of school for the summer. This suited us all just fine, and I was thankful for the opportunity to spend the majority of their summer with them.

I felt a sense of relief also because at our last court hearing, my ex-husband had made negative comments about my working outside of the home, instead of being a stay-at-home mom. Now that I actually *was* at home, I thought that he might ease up on his criticism of me for a change. I was right, or so I thought, because except for the occasional flat tire the night before our court hearings, things were strangely quiet.

Since I was now between jobs, I was free to continue investigating my health problems in an attempt to get a reliable diagnosis and hopefully, a cure for whatever was bothering me. I took advantage of the time the children were in school to visit yet more doctors, and have more tests done, to no avail.

By the end of the summer I began to notice odd things happening to me. I began to count things, a form of obsessive compulsive disorder (also a symptom of Lyme). I would find myself counting buildings as I drove by them, or counting the number of light posts along the roadway. I felt ridiculous, and wondered if this new habit was from the stress or just a sign of an idle mind. In addition, my somewhat random episodes of palpitations and so-called panic attacks seemed to be on the increase.

I arranged to meet with a cardiologist to discuss my new

concerns. He agreed with me that my family history warranted cardiac testing, so I was quickly signed up for a stress test, a heart scan, an EKG, and to boot he had me wear a holter monitor for over a month, in order to catch the episodes of palpitations whenever they might arise.

As it went, I had episodes now quite regularly, and the doctor could clearly see my tachycardia (fast heart rate). I would have a series of beats lasting several seconds to a minute or more, and then my rhythm would return to normal.

I was told that I had an AV node arrythmia, and for about three months it played with me regularly, sending me often to the emergency room because of too slow a heart beat, or forcing me to lay down because my heartbeat was racing. Along with these episodes, I became short of breath and sometimes I would see spots, as can happen just before fainting. I could no longer travel by car, because the episodes came upon me without warning, and making me unable to function in that capacity.

My inability to handle a motor vehicle was probably for the better anyway, as I was now having trouble reading road signs. When I looked at them, they would often appear blank to me, as if there were no words printed on them. Other times I would have to read the signs more than once, as my interpretation of the words upon them kept changing with each glance. "Right turn on red" to me might just as well have read "right turn on Ralph." or "right time for rocks." Driving was becoming confusing and too complicated for me to do safely, and I didn't know why.

As for my tests, the heart portion of the scan was perfectly clear, as was my stress test. Despite multiple areas of attenuation (spots) over my liver, the doctor disregarded them and gave me a clean bill of health. He carefully noted a diagnosis of "stress" in my medical records and offered to give me the name of a "really great" counselor that he had heard of, should I desire to speak with one.

How frustrating it was for me at that time, because I knew I was getting increasingly sick and yet every doctor I saw was convinced that I was inventing my symptoms. Rarely a day went by that I wasn't completely exhausted, and I still had the problems with pain and lack of strength associated with my left side. My balance and coordination were suffering and I kept falling or bumping into things. There were bruises all over my body that I did not remember getting.

After several weeks, the arrythmia stopped as suddenly as it had begun, but following that came another set of problems; new ones that I never in a million years imagined would be coming.

I began to have attacks of flushing, some kind of chemical reaction in my body and tightness in my throat, when eating food. At first the reactions were minor, self-limiting and few and far between. This would leave me to think "what the heck was that?" But then they increased in both frequency as well as intensity; despite my having no known allergies of any kind.

I began to react to lobster and shellfish. Then I reacted to salad dressings and prepared sauces. When the attack would happen, it would be instantaneous and I would feel a rapid flushing sensation, then a wave of a nausea, followed by throat spasms and difficulty breathing. Once in awhile I would have a red patch on the skin of my chest, but that was the extent of the external manifestations. However, the severity of the reactions was what made dealing with them so difficult. After the initial "phase" of the reaction which would last about fifteen minutes, it would be followed up by an incredibly forceful shaking phase.

During this time my heart rate would soar and at one point it was recorded in the over 200 bpm range. This part of the reaction was a lot like riding an adrenaline train. I could not control the shaking, so all I could do was to hang on for dear life and ride it out for however long it lasted. The force of the reactions were directly proportionate to the ingestion of the offending substance, so when they started, I could pretty much tell how bad they were going to be, which did not help matters much except perhaps to lessen my fear of them a little bit.

That phase typically lasted about a half an hour. Once the shaking had ended, the last phase would occur, which included feeling like I was hit by a truck, and I would have to urinate and then sleep for several hours in order to recover.

All during this chemical reaction, my breath would smell foul, I would perspire profusely and become very agitated and argumentative. I had no idea what this reaction was called, nor could I find it in any medical textbook, anywhere. Doctors looked at me like I was crazy when I tried to describe it to them. In the emergency rooms, I was doped up with Benadryl which did nothing except make me more ill and listless while the doctors merely observed what was happening to me, often shaking their heads.

I was diagnosed with anaphylactoid-type reactions, not true anaphylaxis but darned close apparently and I was told to avoid the offending substances and carry an epi-pen.

Since I had no idea what might be causing the episodes, I had no idea where to even begin looking. This was troubling enough as I already wasn't feeling well, but to have to be suspicious of everything that I put into my mouth was a newly found hobby; one that I had no interest in pursuing willingly.

Nevertheless, because the reactions were occurring more frequently now, I decided that the best way to sift through this needle in a haystack was by recording every single food item's ingredients that I put into my mouth. If I was successful eating that food, then all the ingredients listed on the label were put into the "good food" chart. If I suffered a reaction, once I was better, I would go back and record the ingredients of that offending food in order to try to pinpoint the trigger.

Eventually, some common denominators became apparent in my ingredient lists, so I thought I had found the anaphylactic triggers. For the most part, I was right. I was reacting to iodine and annatto, (a yellow plant-based food dye); and shellfish and anchovies. I also reacted to things containing ammonia, like hair permanents or hair dyes, or the smell of baby diapers, believe it or not. I even reacted to pesticides on sprayed fruits and vegetables.

In an attempt to discover the cause of my reactions, I even went so far as to have a small sample of a salad dressing analyzed that I had reacted to. One of my husband's co-workers at his workplace had a wife who was employed at a major food testing laboratory. Her job was in fact, to determine the purity of food ingredients and test for quality control for leading food manufacturers. She smuggled in a bit of the salad dressing for us and on her lunch hour, performed whatever testing she could in order to determine exactly what ingredients might be present in the sample causing my reaction. Ammonia was the one that surfaced unexpectedly and I learned from her that its presence was probably more due to the cleaning solvent residues used on the food processing equipment rather than it being an actual ingredient intended for human consumption.

Knowing what triggered my reactions made eating a little bit easier for a period of time, and that was good because I still was not feeling well, already having enough to handle. The pain in my left side had increased to a level where heating pads and analgesics did nothing for me. There were days also that the cumulative effects of the spasms in my back and shoulder were so forceful that my head literally felt like it was going to explode from the pain. I suffered terrible migraine headaches and talked to a neighbor who also had migraines to see if she had any suggestions about what medications to ask my doctor about. My doctor prescribed Imitrex and something else I can no longer remember, but the medications did nothing to alleviate the pain.

I told my husband that when I had my headaches if I could not respond to him or couldn't answer a question properly to suspect a stroke – that is how horribly painful the headaches were. On those days, I could only spend the day in bed, with the curtains covered to ensure darkness. The muffled sounds of my family behind my closed bedroom door was far too loud for me, and even the sound of my own breathing felt unbearable.

Hospitals could do nothing for me. I thought maybe I had an aneurism. I secretly wished I would have a stroke already or that someone would please kill me and put me out of my misery. Even sleep escaped me during the headaches. I now look back and wonder how I ever functioned at all with the terrible pain I had to endure. There is no way humanly possible to function with that type of pain and I prayed to God that no one else had to suffer the unbearable pain I was experiencing.

Between the horrible migraine headaches and my food allergy problems I surely had enough to deal with, wouldn't you think? Unfortunately, the problems were only just beginning to surface in my life. Thankfully my less-than-ideal childhood and difficult young adulthood had prepared me to be a strong person, as I surely was going to have to draw upon that experience to get through the next part of my life.

One night in August of 2001 while I was tucking in my then ten-year-old son for bed, he suddenly crossed his arms and announced out of the blue that I was "mean". Not knowing what had brought on this sudden change in behavior, I implored him to please talk to me so we could figure out what was troubling him. Out of the mouth of babes came my answer. He told me that his father had told him to say that to me.

After our discussion, I thought to myself that perhaps my ex was up to his old tricks and I spoke with my husband about my son's comment. In a way we both suspected that my ex was performing his usual verbal let's-bash-the-children's-mother-in-front-of-them routine. But in some small manner, the sinking feeling I got from remembering my son's harsh words hit me a bit harder than I expected. Something was amiss. I could sense an impending feeling in my gut, although I did not yet know the cause.

My son continued his acting out behaviors and tried to pick fights with me whenever we were together. This made him difficult to manage at this time of his life, because he was physically growing stronger and I was physically growing weaker. I was ill most days now, and spent the majority of my days holed up on the living room sofa with heating pads on my shoulder, back and/or arm. While each day was a definite struggle now, I certainly was not prepared for the next shock I would receive.

I received a notice of a court motion that my ex-husband had just filed, announcing that he was filing for a change in the custody arrangements under the premise that there was child abuse happening to the children while in my care.

I was absolutely livid at his shocking, and untrue allegations. Suddenly my son's difficult behavior began to make sense. My ex had been prepping him to act up in order to either provoke me into some sort of negative behavior or discipline to support his case, or else he was preparing my son to say negative things about me that were untrue, in order to win a reversal of physical placement of the children.

As if everything I was dealing with was not enough, now I began to be nauseated throughout the day and night time too. I remember wondering what else could possibly go wrong. I also was suffering from horrible menstrual cycles every month and my abdomen seemed to be growing more bloated and painful with each passing day.

I returned to my general practitioner when an appointment with my gynecologist failed to reveal anything unusual. Then I began to have new pain, in my lower abdomen. To me it felt like there was something sitting on my internal organs, and I was incredibly uncomfortable.

To add insult to injury, the new court motion began the process all over again of having to appear in court, having to pay attorney fees, and having to have a new home study done for the upcoming custody trial.

Since I was now accused of child abuse, the pressure was on me to continue to parent in a near-perfect manner at all times, even when I was throwing up in the toilet or walking around with my head in a vice grip. I could no longer discipline my children in any productive manner for fear of it being misconstrued in the courtroom and the children instinctively took advantage of this fact. An effort to try a harmless but creative disciplinary process I had seen on a talk-show backfired miserably when in court my ex twisted the circumstances, and the motivations completely around. No matter what I did for discipline, it was improper in the eyes of my ex-husband, and he would utilize whatever he could, in court.

My current husband, their step-father, also couldn't discipline my children either, because we were both being examined under the microscope that is the family court system. They were looking for *anything* that could be construed as odd or inappropriate behavior towards the children, and yet they were finding nothing at all, but that didn't stop them from looking or microanalyzing our family life.

My health during this time period continued to spiral downward. I could barely function and I was gaining weight at an alarming rate. The unsympathetic doctor told me to go home and stop worrying about my health, so I angrily got a second and a third opinion. Finally, a miracle happened, or I should say an accident happened–sort of a divine intervention, if you will. My ex-husband, in all of his supreme nastiness was utilized in answer to my prayers to discover one aspect of what was medically ailing me.

One evening just before it was my ex-husband's time to pick up the children from our home, it was raining and my son had just returned from a school overnight field trip. He smelled badly and I urged him to take a shower before his father showed up. He flatly refused and we argued a bit. But as young pre-pubescent boys tend to be rather fragrant and in not a nice way, my parental influence eventually won him over, or so I thought, and into the bathroom he went.

As I awaited the familiar sound of the showerhead in action, I called to my son through the closed bathroom door. He replied that he now was *not* going to take a shower because he had (rather conveniently) forgotten his clean clothing.

He wasn't getting off the hook that easily. I told him I would be *happy* to get his clothes for him, and that he should take his shower in the meantime. Well, boys will be difficult boys and when I opened the door a crack to give him his clothes, I tossed the bundle onto the floor so as not to open the door too widely. Unfortunately for me, my son's father showed up outside, honking his horn from the curbside across the street (he never, ever came to our front door–not once in three years).

My son took the opportunity of the slightly opened door to run out of the bathroom, past me, and out the front door, leaving behind his jacket and inhaler. He was needing the breathing device from time-to-time, especially on muggy, ozone-filled days like that evening. I immediately realized that he had forgotten his things and thought that I could catch him before his father pulled away from the curb.

I really did not want to be anywhere near my ex-husband because of his terrible temper and our pending court trial. But I reasoned that maybe just this once he would just *accept* the fact that I had something for our son and be gracious enough to let me give him his things. Unfortunately I was too innocent in my assumptions. Yet with good intentions, I set out in my socks and into the rainy street, to deliver my son's inhaler and jacket to him. My ex was parked across the street and on a diagonal from our doorstep so I had to cross the street in order to get to his vehicle.

When I reached the center of the street, I raised my right index finger in a sign that I had intended to mean "wait a minute". My ex apparently saw this as a sign of confrontation, because he immediately put the car in reverse, and backed it up a couple of feet. Seeing this, I halted in the middle of the street, and said "no wait a second", making a stop sign with my right palm facing him.

Unfortunately for me, he had no intention of stopping. Instead, my ex gunned the engine, put the car in drive and pulled out into the middle of the street, and was headed straight for me.

Since I was luckily only about a car length away from him, I thought quickly and was able to place both of my hands on the front of the hood of the car as it careened into me. I pushed as hard as I could off of my hands and somehow managed to get my lower half of my body and my legs, out of the way of the front bumper.

In the process of doing this, my body twisted around and although I landed on the driver's side of the car on the street in an upright position, I had to hop on one foot to keep from falling down and being run over. In fact the car's front wheels were so close to my feet that I thought they were going to be flattened by the tires.

As the car zoomed past me, my instincts kicked in and my right hand struck the driver's side window once, but not forcefully. I remember saying "Jesus–are you trying to kill me?" I watched my ex-husband blow the stop sign on the corner and continue on his way, leaving me to stand in shock in the middle of the street at what had just occurred. I looked around but there were no neighbors outside who might have witnessed what had happened either, so I was all alone.

As my luck would run, my husband returned from work at that exact moment, pulling his car into the spot behind where my ex had been. I questioned him, but he had not witnessed anything my ex-husband had done, nor had he seen how close I came to being deliberately run over by his car.

I was furious at my ex-husband's behavior however, and suddenly I realized that during my vaulting maneuver over the hood of the car, I had somehow twisted my right leg out of the socket and then back into it again. This hurt a great deal and it was all I could do to limp back into the house, with the help of my husband.

Once inside, I examined my leg in the bathroom, and noticed that it was reddened and swelling. It was painful so I put some ice on it. My husband and I discussed what happened and we made the decision that we should report the incident to the police. (Okay, here comes my so-called criminal history, subject to interpretation).

To make a long story short, the police believed my ex-husband's version of what happened, which was that I had deliberately *thrown* myself in front of his car and that I had been running around *both* sides of his car, pounding on the windows and shouting obscenities at him.

Neither of our children backed up his story about this, and I did learn later from the police report, that the children were never even questioned about the incident. I did discover however, that my ex had told the police a story about how I was *on trial for child abuse* and that he was "concerned" for the safety and welfare of our children.

With this new information, the police asked my children very pointed questions that had already been well-rehearsed at the direction of their father, during the hour-long ride to his home that evening.

The information, later revealed in the detailed police report of the incident, in fact, never once asked the children any questions about the hit-and-run incident *at all*. My ex was never mentioned in the report as having been interviewed either. When the children *were* questioned by the officers, they were spoken to together, and not separately, as is supposed to be standard procedure. Again, they were never once asked about the hit-and-run allegations, but instead focused entirely on the supposed child abuse occurring in my home, convincing the police I was the guilty party by reciting what their father had rehearsed with them, and ad-libbing additional lies in the process.

Some hours later, the local police department contacted my husband and myself, and told us that because I had no witnesses and it was basically three against one, I was to be arrested. I was furious because I had been injured, had not done what I was accused of doing, and I was in fact, the incident's reporting party. During the rest of the evening I kept telling the police that they were arresting the wrong person.

I never had my rights read to me nor was I handcuffed, either. In fact, my husband was free to drive me down to the station himself, and did so, despite my injured leg. I was fingerprinted and had mug shots taken (how humiliating was that?) but otherwise was treated respectfully as I sat in the tank. I was asked several times if I wanted to change my story, but the truth was the truth and I had told the truth. **I was falsely arrested.** I was required to post bail and on condition of release, sign a no-contact order to ensure that I did not contact my ex-husband, the "victim" of the incident; for seventy-two hours.

The idea was humiliating, embarrassing and completely abhorrent to me that I had been arrested for something that my ex-husband had *done to me, and had lied about.* And yet *he* was the one given credence, and once again, (probably because I was female), and due to his ability to lie convincingly, I was ignored.

Throughout the entire process, I remained respectful and calm and kept telling the same story over and over, despite the officers' attempts to elicit a different one from me. "Are you sure you don't want to change your story," they would repeatedly ask me. "No, because I am telling you the truth," was my response each time. The officer would only shake his head, presumably because of my conviction and the fact that he was so convinced my ex had told the truth.In fact, it took about seven attempts for the police to be able to fingerprint me, because the digital machine simply would not work where my prints were concerned. I noted that and said to the police officer, "funny how the machine won't take my finger-prints, isn't it", I said. "Maybe that's because you are arresting the wrong person," I quickly added, in quiet assurance.

Even though no charges were ever filed, I did have to appear with an attorney two days later so he could talk with the district attorney. This required my husband to take a day off of work, as I could not drive downtown Milwaukee because I was too ill.

The DA quickly dropped the case and even my bail money was refunded. But I was technically arrested, and now I was "in the system". I resented that fact because I had not done anything wrong in the first place except to show concern that my son did not have his coat and medicine.

As was expected, my ex-husband immediately took this incident into the family court room, where he and his attorney exploited it fully. They told blatant lies about my emotional and mental health and my recent "arrest".

Despite the fact that no charges were ever filed and the sup-posed arrest was not even considered a crime, my attorney objected to its consideration in the case but the family court com-missioner overruled his objections. This is the point that my ex's attorney made his famous comment that **if the children were allowed to be kept in my care that I would kill them.**

His cruel and ridiculous comments were objected to once again by my attorney, but the court commissioner agreed with my ex and his attorney. I had been arrested, therefore there must have been a *good reason* for it, so therefore I was not setting a good example as a parent. A temporary change of placement order was entered that allowed my children to go live with my ex-husband for the remainder of the summer until school resumed. There was nothing I could do, I had to comply. My ex gloated at his power to destroy my life with his lies, and naturally, I was crushed.

For three weeks after the hit-and-run incident, the pain in my right thigh was unrelenting. I could not figure out if I had torn a ligament or if it was muscle pain that I was experiencing, so I made an appointment with a doctor at my regular clinic, to take a look at my leg. He examined it carefully and then ordered an MRI to be done. A couple of days later, the MRI was completed and I found myself limping back to the doctor for the follow-up appointment.

He asked me questions about how I was feeling, and examined my leg once again. He manipulated it into a bunch of strange positions, some of which were painful and some of which actually offered some relief. By the end of the examination, the pain had ceased entirely (and interestingly, it never returned). I asked for a copy of the report of the MRI to add to my medical records, because I had long been keeping copies of everything done to me in the hopes of finding a "cure" for whatever was ailing me for the previous ten years.

While I sat in his office, I read the MRI report and I noticed that it stated that there was an "adnexal mass" of about 6 cm in size, located on the left side of my abdomen. I asked about the mass and the doctor told me to speak to my regular physician about it. He acted almost nonchalant, as if the growth was no big deal (it was currently the size of an egg).

I made another appointment the following day to talk to my GP. I brought along the MRI from the first doctor and the report from him as well. When my GP inserted the film into the light-box, I saw his mouth drop open, followed by a long silence.

"What exactly is that?" I remember asking him, as I watched him try to comment on the mass he was analyzing. "Well, um, you have a mass–a tumor in your abdomen." The way he said those words to me was almost apologetic, for this was the same doctor I had been visiting over and over, and who had not believed me when I had repeatedly told him that I was not well.

Although he did not apologize for the harrassment he had provided me over the previous months during my office visits, nor did he correct his diagnoses from those visits or the accusations that I should seek counseling from a psychiatrist or a psychologist, he did offer to give me the name of his wife's gynecological oncologist. Oncologist, I thought, that's a cancer doctor.

I said "no thank you" in the kindest way possible, which at that point, because he had missed the tumor and harrassed me in the process probably sounded a lot like a verbal kick in the badoobies; and I angrily left his office.

I cried all the way home, because I knew a little about cancer, and that was something I did not want to have. And yet, in a very small way, perhaps finally having a diagnosis for what was making me so ill was a good thing, because now I had a name for why I never felt well and why I was in so much pain. Gee, I thought, cancer is really an awful thing if it causes migraines, pain, anaphylaxis, disorientation, OCD, and all the symptoms I had been experiencing. I had no way of knowing that it was not the tumor inside of me that was causing the majority of my symptoms, but that it was actually Lyme disease.

By August of 2002, I had my surgery and the now 8 cm tumor was removed from my abdomen along with half of my reproductive system. My left ovary apparently was also riddled with cysts, and the tumor itself had begun to burst, leaking fluid into my abdomen. The oncologist told me that if either the tumor or ovary had ruptured, (and were very close to doing so), that I would have bled to death within a day or two.

Before the surgery I had no way of knowing if I would have cancer or not until after the operation. In the middle of surgery, the oncologist would remove the mass and perform a biopsy upon it while I was still under anesthesia. Only then would the status of the tumor be revealed.

The two-week wait for the day of surgery was painfully slow, and I can fully sympathize with anyone having to go through that process to determine whether they have cancer or not. Tears streamed down my face as I met the surgeon and his young residents just before I went under. I actually thanked them for choosing a career in oncology to help people in my situation. It was tough going into surgery not knowing if you have cancer or not, and I was grateful there were so many skilled hands desiring to help me. Luckily when I awoke from my laparotomy, the recovery nurse was happy to inform me that I was one of the fortunate ones whose tumor would thankfully turn out to be a benign dermoid.

In a way, my ex-husband's horrible anger problems toward me turned out to be a blessing in disguise. It did solve the mystery of my abdominal problems, and even saved my life from a ruptured tumor and ovary. I am in a way, thankful that the process was something I had to go through. But it was unfair nevertheless that the entire situation would be utilized against me in the family court in order for him to get what he wanted. What he wanted was to take the children away from me and my husband, and he would stop at nothing in order to get them.

A day after my tumor surgery, I found myself back in the hospital, because I suffered another bout of anaphylaxis when I tried to eat some processed hash brown potatoes.

Not realizing that the food was causing the problem because I was so dizzy and nauseated, I called 9-1-1 and had an ambulance take me to the emergency room. There a young doctor decided I needed a barium enema to determine what might be going wrong in my bottom end.

Why he came to this conclusion, I'll never know, but I withstood the indignity of that examination by a new Xray technician-trainee, despite my post-surgically bloated belly and my inability to hold

my position due to the pain and sutures making the process difficult for her.

Of course the lower GI Xray was "normal", and I was sent
home with a diagnosis of what basically amounted to gas. (To the
best of my knowledge, gas doesn't cause anaphylaxis guys!)

I spent the next few weeks trying to recover from my recent
surgery. During this entire process of finding the tumor and having major surgery to remove it, the family court commissioner
decided that due to my arrest, my ex-husband and I now needed
to attend family counseling. This after spending the previous
thirteen years together and five more years divorced and not
communicating during any of that time, in the court's eyes, was
going to suddenly solve all of our problems. I thought the idea
rather ridiculous when you think about it, but with all respect to
the courts, whatever is ordered, you must do.

Because of my tumor surgery, I was unable to attend more than
one session of counseling before my operation and then I missed
a substantial amount of sessions following the surgery. I could not
travel, I could not walk around the house, I certainly could not
attend counseling sessions two hours away from my home, so I
called in sick every week.

At first the court commissioner criticized me for my failed
attendance, but when I explained that I had just had major surgery
and more-or-less a partial hysterectomy, she did say "well, I think
you deserve at least 30 days to recover." How gracious of her, I
thought sarcastically. Wasn't anybody going to give me a break?
So counseling was ordered again, this time with two counselors, a
male and a female, and this was supposed to even the playing field
between my ex-husband's lies and the truth.

Counseling seemed like a bad joke, and the joke was on me.
After learning that my ex-husband had a degree in psychology,
the counselors treated him more as a colleague than as a patient
ordered to appear by the courts. Discussions were completely

one-sided and to make matters worse, I was feeling the full effects of the Lyme, the stress, and my recent surgery.

In my fragile state I broke down and cried every counseling session, or else spent the entire time defending myself against my ex-husband's imaginary accusations. I sat there listening incredulously to whole conversations he related that were entirely fabricated. As you might imagine, we made no progress. I was accused of child abuse, I was innocent, and absolutely no one was listening to me.

I stated over and over that I was innocent of child abuse, yet my ex was believed and I sat there accused. Even the counselors told me that they needed to "find out for themselves" whether I had been abusive or not. I told them *that* was up to the *courts* to determine, and that the counselors were hired by the courts to improve communication between my ex and myself.

The sessions made no progress with me excusing myself to go to the bathroom because I was so sick every week, and crying when I wasn't in the bathroom. The counselor's attitudes became dead set against me due to my inability to focus or participate meaningfully. They finally fired us as clients, and then proceeded to testify against me and my "bad attitude" during the trial.

Although they couldn't say exactly what *was* wrong with me, when my ex's attorney volunteered the word "intransigent", one counselor lied and agreed with him that I could have been deemed as such. Not that I *was* intransigent, but she agreed with my attorney that my so-called behavior during counseling could *possibly* be construed as such.

My ex's attorney also took his leading questions a bit further. He next attempted to describe the symptoms of a person with borderline personality disorder, that he read during the trial from out of some psychiatric textbook. He then asked the counselor if my behavior could be interpreted as similar to that of someone with that disorder, and the counselor irresponsibly said, "yes".

Despite the fact that she was not a medical doctor, that she had no ability or authority to diagnose me and had not examined me, she was allowed to testify as an expert witness, and say anything to agree with my ex-husband's attorney. I personally feel she did this out of spite for me because I had refused to answer her questions when our sessions began to fall apart, and I even walked out of the last session due to the complete lack of professionalism exhibited there.

What I found interesting was that during her testimony, the counselor sat nervously upon the witness stand and absolutely *refused* to look at me the entire time she was there. It seemed to me as if she was absolutely aware that she was lying and was afraid of being caught, as if by avoiding my gaze her guilty testimony against me would not be revealed. Even my attorney made a comment about the counselor's lack of professionalism on the stand, but the damage was done and I was now "intransigent" and labeled with "borderline personality disorder."

So now I was being accused of being mentally ill–when all I had wrong with me was Lyme disease and severe stress. I was trying to recover from a major surgery while being forced to travel four hours (round-trip) just to experience the privilege of having my ex and the two so-called objective counselors attack me with accusations of child abuse. I wonder how anybody else would react under those circumstances; and yet I had been far from intransigent.

By the time the trial was well underway, I was recovered from the surgery, but my Lyme symptoms were progressing to the point that I desperately needed medical attention. I struggled to answer questions upon the witness stand and I was accused more than once of being difficult because due to the brain fog, my memory was poor and I had difficulty with my answers. My ex's attorney was rebuked by the judge for yelling at me several times in an effort to get me to answer questions that I struggled to communicate effectively.

At home, the smallest provocations via phone or letter by my ex-husband would send me into an angry or tearful rage, though I was always careful not to exhibit it in front of my children. As I remember it and as my husband told me, I did not have a problem with anger around the kids, at least I was no more angry than any "normal" parent. I was however, argumentative for no apparent reason, and I was rapidly losing my ability to control my thoughts, my mouth or my actions.

When the kids were away and I was free to react as I needed to, things began flying through the air. I remember smashing a telephone following a heated telephone conversation with my ex-husband, who had just refused to honor my visitation schedule yet again, and would not let me see my children. He did this routinely because he knew that I could not afford to file contempt charges each time he pulled a stunt and he exploited those opportunities whenever he could abuse them.

I wanted my children back and I knew that anything I would do would be perceived as negative in the court of law, so I was always very careful to control what now manifested into a very hair-trigger temper. But this day I had no such ability and the phone was one of those wall telephones that didn't work very well anyway. I know you have had one of those phones where every time you talk on it, there is static in the background, you can't hear properly, and every phone call is just plain annoying.

My ex frustrated me so much that after I hung up the phone, I ripped it off the wall. Believe it or not, because the phone was not working well, we had already purchased a replacement phone for it the day before, but had just not yet taken the time needed to install it. So I knew that if I wanted to destroy something, that the phone would be a good candidate. (Yes my mind works that quickly, even in a fit of anger!)

I also had voluntarily gone to counseling in the past during my divorce to help me deal with the difficulties in that process. At one session, I remembered my counselor telling me that one of the best ways to dissipate anger is to take it out on an inanimate object. I had really never tried that before, but today I was having a real problem controlling my temper, so I thought, okay, what the heck. Come on phone, let's have at it.

I took the phone and placed it onto a stool and went and got ahold of a hammer. I pounded the phone to death and every blow I struck I named the things that I was angry about. Blam! that's for your stupid attitude (my ex). Wham! That's for the stupid court crap I have to deal with. Kabam! That's for this stupid illness that is driving me crazy that nobody believes I have.

I purposely and methodically murdered our telephone. When I finished, there were nothing but broken pieces of twentieth-century technology all over the kitchen floor. I realized that what I was doing was actually pretty stupid, but I *did* feel better afterwards, so my counselor's theory had been correct.

I cleaned up the mess and installed the new telephone. The next time the children were at our house, they noticed the new phone and asked me where the old one went. I explained to them, "Mommy killed the telephone" (as a joke), and described what I had done to it and why. Although the children laughed off the incident at the time, later on in court, it would return to haunt me, this time rewritten into something that occurred in front of the children, and supposedly frightening them in the process.

Of course there was never any evidence and it became a he-said she-said battle, but since my credibility had been so carefully and systematically destroyed by my ex and his attorney, guess who always won the argument?

My attorney would later say that "a well-rehearsed lie is more believable than the truth", and he wasn't kidding. I told the truth, and as per usual, my ex lied in court, and everyone believed him. ❖

"A good listener is not only popular everywhere,
but after a while he gets to know something."

– Wilson Mizner (1876-1933)

❖ Chapter 7 ❖

Calling All Experts

Eventually I recovered from the shock of the temporary change in placement. I also knew that if we somehow lost at my upcoming trial, that I would be required to work in order to fulfill child support requirements, so I began to look for work. I didn't really feel very well at this time, but I knew I had no choice but to return to the workforce.

I did manage to find employment and began on September 10, 2001; one day before nine-eleven occurred. I would receive substantially less pay than my previous job, but I was happy working for a smaller company and thought that I would fit in nicely there.

The tragedy of 9/11 occurred the following day and I saw firsthand just how compassionate the upper management of my company was. That was a good thing I would come to discover, and I felt extremely lucky to have found such a great place to work. I was very appreciative of my position because times were tough, good jobs were scarce, and plants were closing all over the country.

I always worked as hard as I could for any employer, but I found myself enjoying my new job mostly because of the fact that these were good people for whom I was working. My intuition about their character would be proven correct, because although I had worked there only a short time, upper management stood by me in complete support while I struggled with my tumor surgery and multiple court appearances.

Once again I missed a considerable amount of time off work due to my illness and court, but because I worked doubly hard when I *was* there, I managed to get my work done and they allowed me to custom-tailor my hours, which was ideal for my situation.

I had been to the doctor several times since my surgery and I was always placed on one antibiotic or another, or I would get a shot of rocephin or penicillin in an effort to stave off some of the effects of my "mystery illness". Because my doctor was the one who had misdiagnosed my tumor, at the very least I no longer had to endure the rigors of his harrassment. Each time I saw him, he projected a new attitude after giving me such a hard time about being ill and missing the cause. Because of this, he now seemed to work a little bit harder to try anything in order to make me feel better, or perhaps, just to placate me and make me go away.

But work became much more difficult for me as days passed. I spent quite a few days working at home while sick, but somehow I always managed to do my job despite feeling awful.

Fatigue was my daily companion, and I suffered stabbing and burning pains in my hands and arm, making typing on the computer very difficult. I wore a brace on one elbow or the other for months at a time due to what was diagnosed as tendonitis, (more likely the spirochetes attacking my joint tissue).

My right knee swelled up and then my left knee would swell. My toe joints swelled. My fingers swelled so that I couldn't wear my wedding ring. My shoulder and arm ached all day long and typing was difficult, requiring frequent rests. To make matters worse, most of my job required me to sit, and my legs would become numb. Still I would try to vary my activities throughout the day in order to work around these problems.

I was terribly stiff and I had trouble remembering what I was doing. I would be working on editing video training tapes and forget what I was doing, repeating tasks I had already completed, or erasing whole sections of valuable footage, requiring a reshoot.

There were many days that I had to pull over when driving to or from work because my panic attacks were so severe that I did not want to have an accident. I would have to wait out the experience until it was safe to continue down the road. It took me longer and longer each day to get to work or get home after work had ended.

My life spun me around like a whirling dervish. I was living a nightmare that I did not know how to explain without anyone thinking I was crazy, so I kept my problems a secret for as long as was humanly possible.

I still suffered anaphylactic reactions from foods, so the safe food choices in my diet were increasingly becoming fewer and farther between. When I'd have a reaction at work, I'd sweat it out in the vacant lunchroom or the ladies' bathroom so no one would see me.

About the time that the trial was winding down, I was suffering from severe stress and my Lyme symptoms were just as bad, no doubt exacerbated by the situation. I cried during work, I cried at home. I was a complete physical and emotional basket-case.

Externally, I had to fight to maintain my composure, feign good health and act like everything was fine. Inside I felt like I was dying. I never felt well, and every morning at work I would hide in the bathroom as long as possible until I felt well enough to sit at my desk. There were days I pretended to be busy working while in the throws of a panic attack. My life was hell and I had no idea why that was so.

The smell of exhaust, machinery grease, solvents and even paint fumes caused reactions while I was at work. Then in April of 2003, the ammonia smell from our blueprint machine sent me to the hospital with anaphylaxis. One day I was at work and the very next day, I had to cease working under physician orders that "something" was causing anaphylaxis. I found myself under doctor's orders to stay home-bound until we could get to the bottom of its cause. This left me feeling terrible about my sudden departure from work, and my employer wondering exactly what the devil was wrong with me.

Just two months later, our trial was over and my attorney had proven that child abuse had never occurred. My children had recanted their lies to their counselors, and even shared with them the information that their father had rehearsed what they were to say to the court officers in order to help him win custody. Bribes of money, shopping trips to the Mall of America and new puppies (believe it or not) were promised in return for their helpful manipulations. Sadly the promises were never kept, and the children felt used, manipulated and heavily guilty for the part they played in the reversal of their living arrangements.

The court ruled that my son was to go live with his father because of comments made by the social worker and the children's guardian ad litem (attorney). Even the elderly judge who had presided over our trial had seemed to be fumbling throughout the entire process.

For example, he couldn't remember that he had criticized my ex-husband during the trial, for his behavior on the stand. He instead said that it had been *me* he had admonished, but he was very wrong. I had sat through an entire three-day trial dutifully taking notes (in between my emergency bathroom breaks) and deliberately not reacting to the lies and manipulations that I heard being spoken all around me. I did this purposely under the advisement of my attorney, who said it would be prudent to present myself in a positive manner during the trial, and I had agreed and complied.

A social worker who admittedly had not done her job due to a death in her family, swore under oath that my face looked "full of rage" when she performed our home study. She accused me of having a flat expression, which she deemed as disturbed or threatening. What she was unaware of however, was that my flat-looking facial expression was a result of the permanent nerve damage resulting from the facial paralysis I had suffered only a couple of years before. **The Lyme-induced neurological damage to my facial expression was the basis upon which she was now discriminating against me.** She legally broadcast her "expert", supposedly well-educated findings and her wrongly perceived interpretations of my offending facial expressions were somehow deemed a reflection of my inability to parent my children.

Additionally, because she had recently had her purse snatched while walking around downtown Milwaukee, she also commented that we lived in a "changing urban environment" (West Allis is a relatively quiet suburb about nine miles west of the downtown area).

Conversely, she stated that the children appeared both "happy and relaxed" while in the company of their father. Obviously impressed by my husband's expensive property, she also stated that his home was in a "beaucolic" area of the state (50 miles away); as if that had anything to do with *his* ability to parent. Upon those comments alone, she recommended a change in placement for both of our children.

The children's guardian ad litem was only slightly kinder to me. Although he said that no child abuse was going on and that he felt I was innocent of those accusations, he did say he felt "something" was going on, but refused to elaborate upon what that *something* was, and suggested instead that I merely had a "full plate."

He recommended that my son go live with his father, and my daughter stay living with me because she could "deal" with my home situation better than my son. To this day I have no idea what he meant by that statement, and he flatly refuses to explain himself, choosing instead to say "that was the past". I say that at the very least, he still owes us an explanation or an apology.

The judge took approximately nine seconds to consider the recommendations of the court officers, shuffled some papers around and then ordered a revision of placement. The judge asked me if I would comply with the court orders, and I said something like "over my dead body am I going to allow you to split up my children. I would rather give up my rights to parent and fight this than allow you to separate them from one another." He peered through his glasses, frowned at me, shrugged his shoulders, and granted my wish. After the GAL made the comment that my statement was the most mature thing he had ever heard from a parent in the courtroom, both of my children were sent to live with my ex-husband.

As the unbelievable verdict was read, I remember feeling like I was going to pass out. I asked my attorney if I was required to sit through the finer points of the visitation arrangements. I do remember that my ex-husband began to cry, probably because he was so relieved that his plan to destroy me had actually succeeded. I tuned out the painful chatter in the background as completely as possible and fidgeted in my chair until it was time to leave the court room.

As soon as I possibly could, I shot out of the room like a race-horse at a starting gate. I didn't bother saying anything to anyone. There was no way I was going to look at my ex-husband's face, or his attorney, or stand around being rational. No doubt the opposition was cheerfully celebrating their deceitful victory.

I nearly passed out as I left the court room. I remember the external room noises sounded muffled to me, as I noticed a loud whooshing sound inside of my head. The people in the parking lot whizzed past me, out of focus. I do remember that I just started walking once I was outside, and I kept on walking until I was nearly a mile out of town.

My husband went to get our car from the parking lot and drove off in the direction I had gone, in an effort to locate me. When he found me, I was in a bit of a daze. My heart was pounding wildly from the unintended exercise and I kept muttering "I do not *believe* this" over and over, under my breath.

I knew if I had stayed in that court room or had been required to speak to anyone, that I would absolutely have lost control. The last thing I wanted to do was to break down in front of my ex-husband or his attorney. But I also did not want to be held responsible for whatever might happen if he decided to confront me either, so I just kept on walking.

After the trial was over, I began to eat less and less, and finally lost my appetite altogether. Some of that was stress, but most of the cause I remember to be that I wasn't feeling well. Nearly every other day I would have reactions to foods and I was completely exhausted from everything I had just been through.

I would eat meat and have anaphylaxis. So I would eliminate that particular kind of meat. I would have a reaction to oatmeal, so then oatmeal was eliminated. Every meal became a fight for nourishment and every food item became the enemy. Eventually, my "safe" food choices became a selection of just five foods. In no particular order, white cheese, saltines, bananas, potatoes and corn became my permanent menu items. I drank water for fluids, and nothing else.

The sicker I became, the weaker I grew, and the more anaphylactic episodes I would experience. Everything seemed to set off reactions, and despite whatever I tried, it felt like my body was rejecting food just because I was so profoundly unhappy.

I wondered if my reactions could possibly have an emotional component to them, but even on good days when I felt a bit better, I would eat food and be fine. The next day I would eat the same food and I'd have a reaction. No, there had to be a physical cause, and I would have to determine what it was. Despite the database of food ingredients I was keeping, I just could not seem to pinpoint the culprit.

During the worst part of what I not so affectionately was calling *the food wars*, I ate only white potatoes and water for every meal, every single day. That practice lasted about a week I think, before my heart skipped a beat so long that I started to pass out. That event sent me to the hospital where it was determined that my potassium levels were far too low. I was also chronically dehydrated, and since I was so underweight I was advised to eat and drink more.

I explained to the ER doctor about the anaphylactic-type reactions, but he just looked at me blankly and called me a "diagnostic anomaly." I was discharged from the ER with instructions to follow up with my primary care physician. Follow up what? My doctor was as frustrated with my body as I was. My doctor threw up his hands and shuffled me off to an endocrinologist.

At least the endocrinologist had the good sense to listen to all that I had been through. When I brought up the subject of Lyme disease however, he replied "we don't deal with that here, we deal with glandular diseases and functional problems." Whatever that was supposed to mean I was not sure, because I thought, *gee, I'm certainly not functioning very well.*

He did perform a series of tests designed to rule out some of the heavy-duty endocrine diseases that are less common. He suspected systemic mastocytosis, adrenal tumors, and a host of things I would not want to attempt to spell. Every test I took returned with what were considered normal results. He called my episodes "spells" and defeated, finally referred me to the Mayo clinic in Rochester, Minnesota.

For anyone who has never been to Mayo in MN, the compound is enormous and very well-run. Like a private club member, you need a referral just to get into the place, but once there, you are treated very humanely and everything is explained to you beforehand. Things run like clockwork and you can really get a lot done within a few days.

Because of the facility's reputation, my husband and I had high hopes for our trip. I was to stay at the clinic for ten days while many expert-level doctors took a good hard look at me in all different areas. If anybody could figure out what was wrong with me, we thought that they would be the ones to do it.

Unfortunately for me however, when I mentioned the word "Lyme disease" to the doctors, they asked me in return why I suspected I had Lyme. I told them it was due to my lengthy medical history and the fact that I had been bitten by a tick and had a rash years before. Because of the 2001 negative Lyme titer that appeared in my medical file, every single one of them ignored my Lyme (self)diagnosis and instead, pursued their own course of diagnostic testing.

I underwent numerous blood tests; and procedures without medication or contrast mediums due to my weird reactions. I even had to endure an upper endoscopy without anesthesia (yucky) for the same reason. I grew very weak from all the testing and repeated blood draws during the ten days there.

When a barium test could not be performed due to an anaphylactic reaction to the barium (a rather inert substance), one doctor shrugged his shoulders, stated glibbly that he had never seen *that* happen before, called one of his colleagues over to watch me shake, and simply cancelled the test.

At Mayo, we were a long way away from our home (a six hour drive one-way), and my husband had to pack food for every single one of my meals; a ten-day's supply, so I could survive the journey. I could not eat food from restaurants, or stores for that matter, because I was constrained by the odd chemical reactions and had to know *exactly* what I was eating lest I suffer one. I remember that I ate only potatoes, corn, white cheese, saltines and baby food bananas washed down with water, at Mayo. I slept when I wasn't being tested or pushed around in a wheelchair by my loving husband because I was too sick to walk.

At the end of the ten-day stint (and another eleven thousand dollars later), the doctor sat with us and explained his findings. "We know this is happening to you. What we don't know is *why* it is happening or how to treat you", he said, giving up on me. "So I'm just supposed to go home and keep not eating to avoid these reactions?" I asked, extremely disappointed at the lack of answers we were given. "Well," he answered, "that's *one* way of handling it." My husband and I, though grateful for the efforts that were made on my behalf, left Mayo more than a little disappointed. I felt like I was dying from starvation and no one cared, not even a huge facility like Mayo.

The honest-to-goodness final diagnosis written in my chart at Mayo was something like, "personal stressors brought about by her ex-husband and family court matters." In reality, I was suffering from chronic Lyme neuroborreliosis, or disseminated Lyme disease.

My husband and I returned home with me literally starving to death and about to enter into the worst phase of my Lyme disease, with little more than unanswered questions.   ❖

❖ Chapter 8 ❖

Meet the Neighbors

By the end of the summer of 2003, our finances were a shambles. My children had already gone to live with their father. My husband was working long hours to try to raise enough money to pay for both our legal and medical bills, but it wasn't enough and I was home-bound, and unable to work. Suddenly we found ourselves on the brink of bankruptcy. We made a difficult decision and sold our house to pay off some of our credit cards that were carrying the bulk of the medical and legal expenses. With the equity in our home, we reasoned correctly that we would be able to find a less expensive home, buy it, pay off some bills, and the burden of living paycheck-to-paycheck would lessen a bit.

We decided also to move out of the city. We had been accused of living in a "changing urban environment" in court and each time I returned home I was haunted by the unkind words the social worker had spoken. My children were no longer around and even neighbors seemed to cast a suspicious eye. Rumors circulated that alluded to the fact that I must have done *something* to deserve the sentence that had been executed upon my family, and our home seemed to no longer welcome us.

What we needed was a fresh start, somewhere as far away from the city as possible. The children had been told by me that if they were sent to live with their father, that things would invariably change, but we really had no idea of the ramifications of those changes. Sadly they were going to find out all too soon, and they weren't going to like those changes either.

We put our home on the market in late September and by Halloween there was high interest in our bungalow. I was becoming nervous because I wasn't feeling very well and my husband's long work hours left him little time to look for a new home. We had years of accumulated furniture and personal items and I did not want to have to put it into storage somewhere. We needed to find a place to live and we needed to find it soon.

To make things harder on me, my eating habits were already a nightmare, and my inability to eat properly weakened me terribly. I was out of breath constantly and slept the majority of the time. In truth, just as I had been wrongly diagnosed many times before, now I *was* feeling depressed due to the removal of my children and the incessant problems with my health. If the anaphylaxis wasn't bothering me, the other Lyme symptoms were.

Now my nighttime hallucinations were revisiting me. There were people in my bedroom nearly every night for a week; and I felt like one of those psychics who talks to dead people. I could talk to these people and a few of them answered me back–so who knows what was really going on. But I knew that they weren't supposed to be there at any rate, and I dreaded going to sleep.

In the meantime, my doctor had the brilliant idea to try to fix my now non-working left arm. He suggested that I put it in a sling during the day to immobilize it. He explained that I must have a permanent tendonitis in my shoulder and that all it needed was rest.

I already walked around the house without the use of my left arm. The idea of a sling didn't bother me too much, because my arm was barely useful at the time anyway. The sling was really just a metaphor for the state of affairs regarding my health, (and life), as far as I was concerned.

My doctor had already tried the immobilization approach with my elbows and my neck a few months before. But I was unable to continue to wear a neck brace because it put too much pressure on my neck, causing terrible headaches–some cure. The arm braces cut off my circulation and I often found my hands go numb, so those were discontinued as well. But I was willing to try anything at this point, for some relief from my pain and health problems.

Having only one arm to use, I let our dogs outside one afternoon, and in doing so, my right hand brushed the wood fence post. "Ouch!" I cried, as I received a good-sized splinter in my right index finger. Since the fence contained chemically treated wood, I did not want to get an infection, so I carefully removed as much of the splinter as I could. However, a small portion of it was still lodged in my skin, but it went unnoticed by me.

Over the course of the next two days, my finger swelled and turned painfully red. I knew an infection was imminent so I went back into the bathroom to try to clean out the remainder of any wood if I could find any. In the next twenty-four hours I suffered terrific chills and felt unbelievably ill. I knew the signs of infection and thought that if I was not better by morning that I would go to the doctor.

The next morning my index finger, now unable to be bent, resembled a balloon more than anything else, making my right hand unusable. Off went the sling from the other arm as I tried to determine which hand was in worse shape.

At the clinic, the doctor removed the splinter and sent me home advising me to soak my finger overnight. He didn't think my chills were significant enough to warrant any alarm at that point. "But I can't bend my finger", I protested.

By the time evening was rolling around, as I prepared myself for bed, I felt violently ill. I couldn't keep warm all evening and put another two blankets onto my bed. Just before retiring for the night, I took another look at my hand to see how it was doing. I noticed an angry purple bruise-like spot that surrounded where the splinter had entered. That is when I noticed the tiny red streaks forming on my hand. They traveled as I watched them, up my right wrist, across the wrist to the underside of my forearm. I was horrified as I watched the front lines of the infection advance in just a few minutes up the length of my arm.

In a very short time, I had grown red lines leading from my finger all the way up my arm to my shoulder. "Oh God, I have blood poisoning," I said to myself and got out of bed. It was now eleven o'clock in the evening and I felt absolutely terrible. I was now visibly shaking from the infection raging inside of me, and I felt very sick, with horrible chills and could not keep warm.

Recognizing septicemia, I knew I had better get to the hospital before the streaks reached my heart. My husband drove me and by the time we got there fifteen minutes later, the streaks had begun to travel over my shoulder and across my chest.

The emergency room hooked me up to intravenous Keflex. I was a bit nervous about trying a new medicine since I had so many reactions to everything. Even following my surgery the previous August, I had trouble with the IV's. What we thought was the saline solution had caused a strong reaction in me. (We later determined it to be a preservative in the solution.)

Now I had to have an IV inserted and as we expected, the saline flush caused a mild, though noticeable reaction in me. The doctor took note of it and the medication was administered any-way, despite the chemical reaction occurring in me from the saline. As the saline flushed the line, my reaction grew worse, adding to my existing problems. The doctor shrugged his shoulders and said merely "wow, that's neat." I didn't feel even remotely neat and was angry with him for not listening, and forc-ing a reaction, but I was hardly in a position to argue.

In the ER, I could not believe how much the medication knocked me for a loop. I felt like somebody had hit my head with a baseball bat and I got a terrific headache. To make matters worse, I became very dizzy and had to lie back. Nevertheless, the medicine was exactly what was needed, because over the course of a few minutes, we watched the red streaks retreat like so many soldiers on a losing battlefield.

The doctor described the cellulitis and septicemia to me and indicated that my choice to come to the ER had been a critical one. Apparently had I gone to bed and waited until the following morning, I probably would not have been here today. As he explained it to me, septicemia is a medical emergency and can be fatal. I was very glad that I had done so much research in medical books, searching for a cause for my physical problems because the knowledge that I gained from doing that just may have saved my life.

After the IV treatment, I returned home with a prescription for oral Keflex to take over the course of the next ten days. I filled it dutifully and began my antibiotic treatment.

The Keflex was not difficult to take, but I did notice that it gave me headaches just like the IV Keflex had done. Not just a mild headache, but a *severe* headache. And during the first three to four hours after taking the medication, my vision would become blurry, I would feel a sort of drunkenness overtake me, and I could not function at all. As each dose increased, the severity of my disability would grow worse. It was almost as if there was something else that was going on inside my body that was reacting to the medication. Well, there was in actuality, but I did not know that at the time.

After five days of putting up with feeling progressively worse, the doctor changed my medication to doxycycline and I took that for two weeks and found myself getting progressively better. An added bonus to the new medication was that some of the pain that I had suffered on a daily basis now seemed to be abated and I was feeling better than I had in a very long time. I felt well enough in fact, that I could now concentrate on finding a new place for us to live.

During the finger infection, our Realtor couldn't attend our open house, so I personally showed our home to a prospective buyer. Realtor or not, I was determined to sell our home and get out of the city, and despite my ongoing infection, I apologized for not looking well and walked the clients through the house. In the end, they made an offer which we accepted and soon we were on our way to finding a new place to live.

I perused the internet looking for a home to purchase. I eventually found one in Fort Atkinson, about fifty miles from where we lived, and located in between two major cities, Milwaukee and Madison. The area was geographically ideal and I remembered that I had visited that town some years before. As prophetically as I had done most of my life, at the time I had said, "I'm going to live here some day." Someday arrived about ten years after my prediction, in December of 2003.

We placed an offer on a run-down ramshackle shell of a house that needed a tremendous amount of repair. Undaunted by the task and grateful that we could actually afford anything at all, we looked forward to the day of closure and a chance to get our finances under some control.

Sadly however, that day never came, as we found ourselves caught in a real estate deal with a homeowner suddenly wanting more money for his property after he had accepted our offer. Through a glitch in the contract, we found ourselves awaiting a real estate lawsuit's final determination hearing, that was scheduled nearly a year away. Now we had a home that we couldn't buy, and a home that was sold and fifteen days to evacuate it.

I scoured the internet to find a home that we could rent, and as luck or fate or whatever would have it, I did find a large enough ranch home for rent on Lake Koshkonong, just outside of Fort Atkinson. Good, we could still move to Fort and be near our prospective home, and we would not have to put our things into storage. The move was ideal. So we'd have to rent for a few months while we waited for the real estate deal to go through, so what. The lake was beautiful and the house, though in bad shape, was good enough for temporary living arrangements.

For some reason the courses of antibiotics I had taken seemed to improve even my constitutional symptoms. I actually found myself able to drive again, which was critical because someone now had to travel back and forth to the new house to handle the move. I ended up being able to pack the smallest boxes into our van and travel down to Fort in the morning, unpack the boxes and return back to Milwaukee. The trips were grueling for me in my condition, but somehow I managed to make them.

Eventually we were moved into the rental home. Immediately I noticed that the dishwasher wasn't connected and the kitchen sink leaked terribly. But a bucket under the sink and a bucket under the drain hose in the basement handled those issues. There were holes in the wall all over the house, and missing tile in the bathroom floor where somebody had attempted to be a handyman but had failed miserably. In the basement, one of the rooms leaked when it rained, causing it to be unusable for storage, and requiring me to mop with every downpour to prevent seepage into the adjoining living spaces. When the dishwasher or sink was utilized, a terribly foul smell would emanate from the basement drain.

The home was perched on the edge of a gulley, on two acres, which were heavily wooded. The trees were beautiful and I tried hard to overlook the home's shortcomings. There was an enormous garage on the property as well, where the overflow of possessions and garage items made their home. The garage was spider-filled, damp and mildew-laden however, so I had to keep watch over the furniture and ventilate the garage on a daily basis so as not to have mold ruin our belongings. The day we moved into the home I found myself back in the hospital due to an accidental injury, so at least I now knew where the medical team could be found if I needed them.

Our landlords were a mismatched couple of folks that seemed nice enough. The man had recently survived a horrific abdominal surgery that had gangrene removed. The woman was a nurse at the local hospital, and as it would happen, also someone who had struggled through a divorce and also had her children removed from her care thanks to her ex-husband. However we had found this couple, we were in good company I suppose, because they seemed to have just about as many problems as we did.

Despite the house's shortcomings, we would manage to stay there, renting month-to-month, for a total of eight months. The inconveniences were rental living at its worst, I suppose, but I was grateful to have found a place for us to stay in the middle of winter. Living among the stacked boxes, all of us were going to be very glad when the time finally came for us to move out.

My son's bedroom walls were painted a ghastly purple and had paint streaks across them that a blacklight could illuminate, which he hated. My daughter was thankful that her room was a bit more normal looking. I was merely glad our baby grand piano fit into the living room along with the other furniture. In the basement all of the boxes that contained our possessions that weren't absolutely critical to daily function were stacked floor to ceiling in two separate rooms. Every closet was jam-packed to capacity, with our packed belongings.

The dogs were required to stay in a kennel in the basement due to the lack of room in the house. The cat made do perched high upon the new living arrangements and the three bird cages were relegated to a back room. I even set up a small fish tank on the kitchen counter to temporarily accommodate our aquarian friends. The tiny home was literally stuffed to the roof with furniture, boxes, people and animals. At Christmas, we stacked furniture in order to make room for our Christmas tree.

Still, the days at the house were peaceful enough. Since I could no longer sleep normal hours due to my illness, I spent many nights sipping hot chocolate and peering through the moonlit back yard, watching the forest animals perform their nightly rituals. Deer, raccoons, wild turkeys, and other wonderful creatures were just a few steps out the back patio door and I enjoyed the ability to nature watch from the relative comfort of the kitchen chair.

I still was not working due to my illness and sensitivities to chemicals and foods. I tried to eek out a bit of a living hawking antiques and collectibles on the internet. Anything I could do to help our finances was a welcome effort. We now had a real estate attorney we had to pay for, a house sitting waiting to be purchased, a family court trial that had gone horribly wrong (and we were now in the appeals process), and medical and legal bills that were escalating. The pressure was enormous on my husband to earn enough money to keep us afloat, and I wanted to help out any way I possibly could.

The business, if you can call it that, in the end, earned very little money. I paid more in postage and selling/listing fees than I received for all the trouble that it was worth. So I abandoned the activity because it seemed like such a waste of time. In the end, I did trade a few of my unwanted possessions for new ones that I at least liked better. I did make perhaps a couple dollars of my own, but the hours required typing at the keyboard proved to be too much for me physically.

I did manage to make friends in the new town, which was good, because we intended on living there permanently. I frequented the post office to mail my packages for the few items I sold and I was becoming friends with the clerks there. I also spent some time in the local library and bank, and I made key acquaintances there who would help me further along on my life path, though much later in life.

My illness, which had been strangely quiet for months after the course of antibiotics from the finger incident, now began to rear its ugly head again. The accident that I had when moving into our rental home also seemed to aggravate my gallbladder problems that had surfaced way back in 1994. I began to again have excruciating pain in my upper right quadrant of my abdomen, and I needed to see the doctor, and soon.

As bad luck would have it, another medical procedure would become necessary. I had to have a papida scan done, to check my gallbladder function. Since I was technically reactive to iodine and contrast media, I could not ingest the fluid that I was supposed to drink. Instead I was given a container of heavy cream to drink, and a radioactive isotope tracer doo-hickey was injected into my arm. The long and short of it was that my gallbladder had ceased to function which caused my pain, and it was now scheduled to be removed.

Okay, so I had to have another abdominal surgery and another organ removed. At this point in my life, I think I was on my ninth surgery, so I well knew the drill. At the hospital I carefully explained as intelligently as I could that I had *some* kind of illness that the doctors couldn't explain, that reacted to various substances (and I gave them the long list). Everyone took note of my claims and away we went into the surgical suite.

After the surgery, I had tremendous problems recovering from the anesthesia. I felt perpetually drugged and it took honestly a couple of months before I was well enough again to venture outside of the house. During that time, my symptoms worsened. My left arm was once again useless, and my balance and coordination were rapidly declining. On top of that, I kept having episodes of vertigo and dizziness and I could barely see sometimes; my vision was a blurred mess, depending upon the time of day.

My gastrointestinal tract was a nightmare, and I had a couple of hallucinations again where I would think I saw someone walking past the doorway. But it would not be indiscriminate people I had never seen before. For example, I saw a person who I had known in life but who was now *dead,* walk by a doorway, smile and wave hello. Now I really began to wonder what the heck was going on.

I was alone in the middle of nowhere. Sure, we had neighbors. They would come out on the weekends. These were lake houses;

vacation homes with few permanent residents. I was surrounded with trees, not human beings. Well, I did see some of those, but I knew that they weren't really there and I was too afraid to tell anyone but my husband about them.

My husband commuted to his job, fifty-two miles away, every day. Because of his long drive, it took him at least an hour to get home every evening. Home alone, I had literally no one to help me in case of an emergency. This was a very rough time for me, as my illness was beginning to hit me full force.

As my balance deteriorated, I could no longer easily drive my car. I spent the majority of my days on the couch, sleeping, reading (when I could see), or looking out the kitchen's sliding glass door at the forest.

My new doctor took a long look at my very painful neck and shoulder and declared the necessity for physical therapy (oh no not again). I was to go twice a week into town, which was just barely close enough that I could drive there, even on my bad days. I was to endure another round of someone manipulating my movement-resistant muscles and frozen neck and shoulder back into motion.

At this point, I could no longer turn my head to the left, or look up or down either. I could not lift my left arm above my head, and I suffered painful muscle spasms and involuntary twitching all day long. I couldn't wear a bra because even that aggravated my condition.

The skin on my back, neck, head and arm was horribly painful to the slightest touch. I couldn't decide what part of my illness was worse, the inability to move, the pain, the hallucinations or the eating problems.

The physical therapist, though well-meaning, was aggravating my condition. First I was placed on some sort of device where essentially you are stretched a little bit at a time. It felt like a human torture device, similar to an ancient stretching rack. When

I was strapped into it, I felt much like I was being hanged, but in the prone position. I thought the device much too dangerous for my tastes. I saw lots of stars after that exercise and said there was no way I was going to go back onto that machine, as I had images of my neck snapping in two.

I already had problems with the cervical disks in my spine, up near C-5 through C-7. I had injured my neck during high school gymnastics practice when I fell from the uneven parallel bars. I had suffered a compression fraction that had apparently healed for nobody ever knew it until many years later. In hindsight, I was very lucky I had not been paralyzed. But when I had to fight with my mother to be able to join the gymnastics team in the first place, I was not about to report any injuries lest I risk being forced to quit as a consequence.

Over the years the disks had deteriorated to the point that one of them was pushing on my spinal cord. It was noted in my medical records that the disk was pushed forward, and was about 40% out of alignment. I wonder now how much of my "pain in the neck" has been due to the old injury that had long since healed; and how much of the pain has been caused by the deterioration of the soft tissues and joints being attacked by Borrelia burgdorferi.

A few weeks of physical therapy did nothing to help my situation again and merely contributed to more suffering. I begged my doctor to cancel or modify his game plan, and we again halted therapy.

Because I could not really travel anywhere, I was left with the majority of my day home alone. On days that I had any energy at all, to help pass the time, I would sometimes take the dogs for a brief walk into the woods behind our house. They greatly enjoyed the exploration, though it was taxing on me.

Several times upon returning, I would notice a tiny bug crawling on my shirt. I would quickly brush it away, but not before I determined that it was a deer tick. The woods were heavily infested with them and I took to inspecting myself and the animals after our walks. I actually found four adult ticks within a period of just three days and decided to keep well away from the woods after that.

I should have looked a little more closely at the tiny critters that had stopped in to visit me. Had I done so, I would have realized that they were part of the universe dropping hints upon me in an effort to reveal the secret of the illness that had evaded me for so long. But I could not really see what was quite literally, right in front of me, at least, not yet.

I did spend a lot of time thinking and observing the creatures in the woods. I was entertained the day a reddish fox galloped along the edge of the curb as he made his way down the street. I had never seen a fox in the wild before, and it felt exciting to me. The wild turkeys that frequented the back yard were also delightful to observe. I envisioned what life must have been like a hundred years ago in our part of the state. We were just up the road from ancient Indian burial mounds and I would visualize the fauna and the very different way of life back then.

At the end of the evening just before dusk, I would often go outside to witness the sun dancing along the rim of the lake just before disappearing from view. One evening I made my way outside in anticipation of the beautiful sunset. As I stepped out the side door, I heard a sound that I had never heard before. It sounded similar to that of a cicada, though it was much lighter in tone, almost musical. I walked around to the rear of the house, and the noise grew significantly louder.

I looked up into the treetops and realized the sound was coming from them. The source of the commotion was the sound of billions or perhaps even trillions of tiny insects gathered together and singing in unison. The sound was beautifully musical and the notes sent a chill down my spine. It sounded to me like the forest was singing, and in that moment, I felt a tremendous peace and tranquility like I had not felt in a very long time.

As I listened to the singing forest, I felt humbled by the spectacular orchestration that was occurring some twenty or thirty feet above me. In that moment I realized how beautifully simplistic nature truly was. If mankind could only be more like nature, I thought to myself. Nature doesn't ask questions, it does not require any answers, it quite simply, *is*.

I think the lesson in that moment for me to learn was the appreciation of simply being in the moment. Not seeking, not asking, just being. The patience of listening, the joy of feeling the forest alive with life and the suggestion that if mankind would only work together in unison as the forest did so naturally, the world would be a much more beautiful place in which to live. While the singing forest would become my motivation later in life, for now, its sweet music felt soothing to my troubled soul.   ❖

Chapter 9

No Kidding

Eventually our real estate deal had its day in court and although we won the countermotion against us, we lost the home on a contract technicality, which left us without a place to move to. I had watched in dismay as the attorney costs for the real estate lawsuit began to chip away at the meager profit we had made selling our previous home. Now we had very little money left, and it might not be quite enough to purchase another home.

It was nearly spring and the thought of having to stay in the ramshackle home any longer sent a chill up my spine. There was no way we could stay there much longer, the smell of the septic gas coming into the house was unbearable. In addition, the landlord and his lady friend were fighting and rumor had it that the house was soon to be sold. We would be out on the street if I could not find some place for us to live, and soon.

As it happened, I spent some time on the internet, searching various neighborhoods, to no avail. Every home I found was either much too expensive or it wasn't large enough. In addition, it was now the month of March, and the selection of homes on the market were few and far between. I did not know how we were going to provide the down payment for the new home, but I really didn't care about that yet; I had to get us out of there no matter what it took.

Eventually I decided to take a look at duplexes. I reasoned that perhaps they were selling more cheaply than single family homes, and as it turns out, I was correct in my assumption. Luckily I found a beautiful, one hundred year old brick victorian "duplex" that was for sale, but it was located in a town forty-two miles north of where we were living. Despite that, I loved how the home looked, or rather could look, with its stained glass windows and large front porch. It was the house I had always dreamed of owning, and here it was, looking right at me.

I talked to my husband about the increased drive to his work place, because I was concerned about his commute. But when it came right down to it, the drive to the new home was actually ten minutes shorter than the drive he currently undertook each day, just in a different direction.

The other issues to consider of course were the children and my ex-husband. Although it was a good idea to put as many miles between our two residences as possible to minimize his stalking behaviors, I knew that the increased distance would be hardest on the children. Unfortunately, we really did not have much of a choice at that point. No other houses were available on the market that we could actually afford. We decided to put in an offer on the duplex, which was really a single family home that had been converted by adding a doorway at the top of each stair-case (there were two of these).

The house was currently in probate and it had been a rental for nearly sixty years, so you can imagine that there were quite a few repairs to be made. In addition, there was mildewy carpeting, damaged suspended ceilings, water damaged walls from leaky pipes, outdated lighting and barely a kitchen on either floor. Immediate renovations would be required, but because the house was cheap, and had character and good bones, we looked past the uglification factor and placed an immediate offer.

The month we placed our offer had produced a record amount of rain and the day we looked at the home, the basement was completely flooded and there was rain pouring into the attic roof courtesy of various holes. Despite this, essentially the home was quite salvageable.

To make our purchase easier, my friend the banker told us about a unique opportunity for which we qualified. Instead of twenty-percent down on the home, the bank only required that we put down five-percent, as the home was technically an owner-occupied duplex. That opportunity was unbelievably coincidental, because five percent was *exactly* what we had left in our savings. The powers that be helped us on that one, and we soon moved into our "dream" home.

As you can imagine, my ex-husband was not exactly thrilled that we had added an additional forty-two miles to the visitation exchanges. However, in the past, he always willingly split the distance in half with us. Because we were ordered by the court to perform the transfers at a police station, (I was apparently dangerous), we chose a town at the midway point to transfer the children.

With this new move, my ex suddenly decided that I had placed an "undue burden" upon him (another fifteen minutes total drive time), and he wasn't planning on driving any farther to get his children. In retaliation for our move without his consent, he filed yet another court motion complaining about our move. On the stand, I was actually admonished by the judge for failing to find a house "anywhere else in southeast Wisconsin" instead of the one that we had purchased. Like we really had a choice–no money, no homes on the market, no time to lose, and according to the judge, we now also had no right to live wherever we wanted to.

I was forced to drive the greater distance, or I should say my husband was forced to do so, because I could no longer drive that far. Fortunately he did this without complaint, though I could not accompany him to pick up the children. He would leave from his workplace in order to do so. He'd first drive the hour-and-a-half to my ex's hometown to pick up the kids, then drive an additional hour-and-a-half to our home.

The drive was not hard on my husband (or so he claimed), but it *was* hard on the children. Still, they did their best not to squabble and instead, found things to do to entertain themselves during the long drive. They also got to know their stepfather more intimately during these voyages.

Before the trial, I had tried to warn the children that if they told the court they wanted to go live with their father, that things would change drastically. I just had no idea that the changes would include forcing them to endure longer car rides in order to get to our new home. I guess the lesson for them was to be careful what you ask for, because the consequences might not be what you expect them to be.

While we were still at the Fort Atkinson rental home, I had begun to notice that my children's attitudes were becoming very negative. To counteract this, my husband would take the children on bike rides around the lake, which they enjoyed. I usually could not go with them because I did not have the strength. But I would watch them have their fun and when they returned, they would tell me all about their adventures.

The rest of the time the children did not get along very well. To me it seemed at first to be due to their age difference. When kids become teenagers they begin to distance themselves from one another. I had experienced that when I was growing up, for I had three brothers. But as I looked more closely and really listened to their conversations, I could see that there was real negativity in their voices.

My daughter treated her younger brother with a new disdain and he retaliated by causing trouble just to annoy her. This activity was something that they routinely had *not* done when they were in my care. To me it seemed as if there were suddenly no boundaries and they certainly seemed to have respect issues between them.

I wondered what kind of environment they were living in over at their father's home. I remembered all too well his lack of involvement in their early years when I was married to him. I had no idea what kind of a substitute parent his live-in lady friend was, but from what my son had told me about her, she lacked even fundamental parenting skills that I felt to be essential, which was not good in my book. In addition, both of the children had kindly informed me that she often swore at them, calling them demeaning names I would never dream of using. When she couldn't control them, she would tearfully slam her door to escape them, telephone their father and complain about "his" children's behavior, often threatening to leave.

The truth was, the barriers between right and wrong, lies and truth, and good and bad behavior were breaking down, at least at their father's house. I caught the children swearing and lying, which was something I never tolerated when they were in my care. But now they "slipped" every once in awhile, and I did not like what I was seeing.

Now practically every weekend they came to visit us, I would have to spend an inordinate amount of time undoing the bad habits that were forming over at dad's house, which was frustrating to me.

In addition, their hygiene habits had literally hit the dirt. They no longer showered, combed their hair nor even brought clean clothing with them. They would attempt to wear the same clothes all weekend if I would let them. It wasn't just a teenager thing, it was a their-father-knows-no-better thing. My ex dressed like a slob and had horrible personal hygiene habits, and he was letting our children behave in the same manner as he did.

My son was angry and hostile toward his sister and mouthy towards me and my husband, which needed correction nearly every weekend, filling our visitation time with dissension. Adding to his frustrations, he was not feeling very well and it was obvious to everyone. My son had complained most of this life about bone pain, joint pains, and his back hurting. He also had problems with his knees. Sometimes his hands or his legs would go to sleep. In addition, he had headaches and he slept inordinately longer than seemed necessary.

He was shorter in stature than most children his age, and it bothered him a bit. In the mornings, he was grumpy most of the time and he had a hard time going to sleep during normal hours.

He had repeated bouts of conjunctivitis in one eye, as did I, but because his hands were usually dirty, I thought it was related to not washing his hands. All of his symptoms were somewhat vague but present nonetheless, but I never connected them with the multitude of health problems that he had endured when he was an infant.

Now however, his attitude had taken a turn for the worse. It took barely a word to set him off and he would throw incredibly dramatic temper tantrums. This was very unusual for him, because he was normally quite a mature and rational young man. But as he hit puberty, we were afraid to cross him because he would explode into irrational anger.

Sometimes he would throw things across the room, or punch his sister. Often he would act like he was three years old and absolutely refuse to budge, laying on the floor in the fetal position as if someone was beating him to death. I caught him more than once actually banging his head against the wall in a harmful expression of his anger and frustration.

This behavior was very different from that which he exhibited when he lived with me. I did not know how to deal with these personality changes, but I did the very best I could, while silently hoping he would soon grow out of them.

When he was reticent, I urged him to talk to me. Then he would unload things that were troubling him by opening the floodgates of his emotions. This usually happened when we were alone, late at night and he could get some quality one-on-one time with me. During that time, he was mature, thoughtful, introspective and extremely articulate. That was the side of my son that I knew and enjoyed and of which I was proud. But the behavior that he was now exhibiting was crossing the line of acceptability and it was very hard for him to control.

It was almost as if there was something else affecting my son, something medically wrong with him. He did not have to say

"I'm not feeling well," I could tell just from his behavior when he was having a good day and when he was not. I altered his nutrition and removed as much sugar and garbage food from his diet as possible. It seemed to improve his attitude in the short-term, but always he would revert to his old behaviors. No, there was something else going on, and I knew it but I could not put my finger on what that something was.

About the same time that my son was having behavioral changes, my daughter, extremely unhappy with the court-appointed living arrangements and my choice to keep the children together (and forcing her to live with her father), began to withdraw into her room.

During visitation in the past, she would play games with us, talk to me and take part in family activities. But now she was sullen, moody, and depressed. She no longer cared how she looked, whether or not she bathed, and she even wore the same clothes as long as she possibly could. My children were becoming clones of their father and copying his unhealthy habits.

In addition to that, because she was so introspective, she refused to talk to me. I am certain that some of that pulling away is natural for a girl her age, because I had done that myself when I was a teen. There was something more happening with her too. She always appeared to have dark circles under her eyes and she slept many more hours than she should have. She complained of headaches and stomachaches and even menstrual problems.

She gained about twenty pounds just in the first few months she went to live with her father, and she was always tired. I encouraged her to exercise more and eat better when she was with me, but her eating habits were horrible and I knew that no matter what I did when she was with me, she would revert back to her old habits as soon as she left.

She seemed to carry a black cloud of gloom and doom over her head and I urged her to do more things with the family. One of those activities was bicycle riding. Both of the kids liked to do that, and they would take bike rides whenever the weather permitted.

On one such trip while she was out riding around, I happened to walk past her room and I noticed a pile of papers on her bedroom floor. Because she spent a good portion of her spare time drawing and she was very talented at it, I was curious to see what she was working on.

Unfortunately for me, what I found was not what I had expected. I examined the drawings before me. They were beautifully depicted caricatures of herself, and her brother. In the pictures, she was sobbing, as if heartbroken. In one picture her brother, a cartoon character with clawed feet (no doubt a statement on aspects of his behavior), had his arm draped around her sobbing character in a sign of empathy and comfort.

The images were so grief-filled that it broke my heart to see them. I knew then that my daughter was carrying a tremendous burden and this was just one form of venting it. I dug deeper into her portfolio and I came across a poem about a character she called a fish-mouse. The poem revealed to me a story about an imaginary creature that, through lies, had forced circumstances in his life to change in a regrettable way. The moral of her story was something to the effect that if you leave things alone and let them be, everything will go as they are supposed to. But if you try to force change, that those changes will not always be good and they may even be something you might regret.

My daughter was expressing her feelings of responsibility toward the lies she had told, and the part she had played in the family's custody reversal. Now her self-criticism and guilty conscience was weighing heavily upon her.

I decided that I would have to find a way to talk with her about the past, and let her know that I understood her guilt but did not agree with it. She and her brother were not to be blamed for what had happened to the family. They had been lied to and manipulated, with promises of money, gifts and vacations by their father just so that he could get what he wanted, in order to hurt me.

I also decided to photocopy these works of art, because I wanted to examine them further in private, as I was certain she would return home any minute and I was not yet ready to confront her.

That evening I did my best to open the door of communication by bringing up the subject of her artwork. She didn't want to talk about it and was embarrassed that I had seen what she had drawn. I assured her that I was not holding her responsible for the family's situation, and she even seemed a little bit better after the conversation.

But now that we had finally moved into our new home, I saw my child increasingly withdraw from civilization. There were neighbor girls who were approximately the same age as my daughter, but she expressed barely any interest in meeting them or "hanging" with them.

My child became a loner, and except for a few friends that remained back in West Allis, she had no one except for her brother, as a friend. This did not sit well with me, for anyone who knows me knows that I like people, and I tried to engage her in conversation with the neighborhood girls whenever they were around, to no avail.

Both children loved to utilize the computer, and the internet was a common stomping ground for them. I like to think that I am a responsible parent, so I invested thirty dollars in parental spyware that records internet usage in a secret place on the hard drive so you can keep an eye on your children's computer activities.

Neither of the children knew about the software, but I didn't spy so much as I kept a reasonable watch over the kinds of sites they were visiting. After one weekend visit, I perused through the sites they had frequented that day. I came across an internet site that my daughter had visited where you post on-line, poetry, prose and artwork for the world to see. I cannot name the internet site here due to any ramifications that may arise, however, it was not as mainstream or widely known as some of the other sites you now read about in the media.

Because of the software program, I didn't even need a user name or password to access the visited sites, even if they required one. It offered me instead, a back-door approach into viewing their files, and I viewed. What I found simply amazed me. As I read further, my curiosity turned to dismay. My daughter was posting very negative thoughts, feelings and statements on a very public forum, the internet. She was doing it, at least until that very moment, without my knowledge.

Her posts went far beyond the typically angst-filled ramblings of a normal, venting teenager. What I found instead worried me immediately. Her artwork and poetry was very dark, even morose. She had designed Manga-style cartoon characters that supposedly represented a comic book that she was working on, yet they more closely resembled herself, her brother and the important people in her life.

As I followed her activities that had been occurring over the past month, I noticed a common theme throughout them. She seemed fixated on Japanese culture, but more precisely, on the ancient Samurai practice of Seppuku, or ritual suicide by disembowelment (also called Hara-Kiri). The grisly process is basically death-instead of dishonor by gutting oneself in the stomach with a special knife, and then being beheaded by a trusted friend. Fortunately to my knowledge, the practice has long been abandoned.

At halloween that year, she desperately had wanted to sew an outfit so that she could trick-or-treat as a Samurai warrior. Because at the time I did not have knowledge about her internet postings, I thought "oh how cute, she's getting into foreign culture," and took the opportunity to teach her how to sew and also to actively *do* something with her.

We worked hard for a couple of weeks on a completely authentic Japanese costume. We made a Haori (kimono robe), with a happi (a coat worn underneath her Haori), a hakama (divided pleated pants that tie at the waist), and a pair of white tabi (socks with a divided toe). She even bought authentic shoes and an umbrella to complete her outfit. (Samurai's used umbrellas?)

But now that I was reading the prose and storylines of her postings, I was having second thoughts about promoting her interests in this new hobby. Clearly she was applying her life experiences to her artwork, which in itself is not a problem. But her journeys on the internet did not have such clear limitations. Slowly but surely she began to cross the line of fictional credibility, and tangible proof of the depth of her despair became disturbingly apparent.

Poem after poem appeared, each one more vibrantly depicting the theme of death and suicide than the last. She likened her thumb with the blade of a knife and longed to drive it into her belly, and end the tremendous dishonor that she felt.

The comic morphed into a description of her fears, her wishes and her own admission that she felt as if she was losing her mind. As I read from day to day, I watched my child describe to me symptoms that a normal person would question might be coming from a person who had a mental illness. Now I was becoming very worried indeed.

I tried in vain to communicate to her about my concerns with this web site. In order to speak with her about it, I had to reveal that I had "stumbled" upon her work. I had no choice but to run the risk that once exposed, she might cease posting and go underground with her activities. At least this way I could monitor what she was doing, to keep an eye on her. In retaliation for my concern, she posted online criticisms of me, and her friends told me in no uncertain terms on their own sites, what they thought of my supposed spying. From my point of view, I was only parenting my child and trying to determine what was going through her mind, but in her viewpoint, I was the enemy, and my supposed wrongdoings were openly criticized in this public forum.

Undaunted, I read on each day and though she suspected but could not confirm if I was still reading her postings, she publicly threatened me with permanently cutting off her love for me (yeah right) and the like should I continue monitoring her. I continued monitoring her for her own good.

Her writings were troubling not only because of the suicide-guilt-dishonor theme, and artwork that colorfully reflected that outlook, but because she was describing things that showed a person without a clear perception of herself in reality.

What I mean by this is that she would describe dreams she would have and then seem confused as to whether or not those dreams were real or if they were only her imagination. She would "forget" whether she had dreamed a thought or only day-dreamed.

Her dark thoughts haunted her both during the day and at night. She was having trouble sleeping, experiencing nightmares about killing people, where she would intimately describe how it felt to murder, down to vivid dipictions of the color of the blood drops. She would look into the mirror and hallucinate that her face was morphing and she would honestly wonder if she was still in reality. To me that was very alarming indeed, and she even openly stated that she wondered whether or not she had a mental illness.

I know now that her nightmares and some of the symptoms of her depression and confused thinking were probably manifestations of Lyme disease attacking her brain. But since she had not yet been diagnosed, there was no way for me to know what was happening inside of her head. If I had known that Lyme was very much to blame for much of what she was expressing, then I could have treated her appropriately. But sadly because that diagnosis was still a mystery, I was unable to put two and two together and figure out why she was behaving so badly.

I continued to watch her on-line antics over a series of months.

During that time period, I contacted her father through letters because he always automatically hung up the phone when I attempted to call him. In the letters, I was careful not to get too wordy, but I stressed the importance of what I felt. I asked him to take our children into counseling due to the lies they had told and because I saw marked depression in both of the children. As expected, my ex-husband purposely ignored me. He didn't even reply to my letters. The children would however, kindly inform me that he mocked me upon receipt of my concerns.

I attempted to find a counseling center that had hours that coincided with my practically nonexistent visitation schedule. I could not find anyone within my geographical region that had Saturday hours that was close enough for me to struggle to drive to. And my husband's taking the children to counseling was out of the question, due to his mandatory Saturday work schedule.

I next tried in vain to get the school counselor and the principal involved in the process. The counselor listened to my concerns about my children's emotional health, especially my daughter's, then quickly dismissed those concerns and left on maternity leave. I called back and reiterated the circumstances to the substitute counselor, but she too, had no interest in providing any counseling to my children, identifying herself as merely a *substitute* counselor.

I talked to the principal again and asked if there was anyone at the school that my daughter, the more depressed of the two, could talk to on a one-on-one basis, or if he could recommend anyone for her to see. The request was stone-walled and ignored. I was told that it was not the school's responsibility to provide *that* kind of counseling, only college or career choices, to my children.

I pressed on with my request. I told them "but you *can* watch her closely and keep an eye on what she is doing". In the end, the principal told me that because my daughter was a straight-A student, that she flew "under the radar" and that because of that, she was not really a concern to him. In his rationale, as long as a student was making good grades, they were not a problem.

Well, I disagree. I say that if you have a student in your school, as a parent, I am trusting you to keep that child safe. If my child is expressing a curiosity or an overt interest in suicide and things of that nature, it is your responsibility as a school principal, teacher or counselor, to do everything in your power to protect my child.

Having said that here, I felt like I was talking to a brick wall. Everywhere I turned, no one would listen to me. My ex ignored me. The school principal said it wasn't his problem. The guidance counselors did not want to help out. I did not have a counselor available on my time with the children. I felt completely at a loss to do anything. My ex did not go to church, so there was no clergy that might have been helpful to her. I could not talk to her friends' parents, because I now did not know who or where they were.

My ex did everything in his power to isolate me from my children, including training them to give out as little information to me about their life and friends as possible. I pulled teeth every time I saw my children to get even basic information about their lives. I was allowed no part in the selection of their high school curriculum nor many other rights one would expect to have as a custodial parent.

Despite some people's ideas (even well-educated professionals), that parental alienation does not occur, I submit to you that it indeed *does occur,* and my ex is an expert on the subject and very effective controlling our children.

I contacted the county social services department and tried to get them to investigate my ex-husband's home and our child's activities there. I told them briefly that my daughter was involved in posting things on the internet that were not appropriate. I could not elaborate fully because I did not want to reveal the serious nature of what I was reading, but I did express enough concern that they should have followed through on my allegations.

Months later I would discover that they had not even recorded our phone conversation in their records. Social services had once again, let my children down by lending me absolutely no credence whatsoever to claims that something was very wrong at my ex's house and that my daughter might be headed for serious trouble.

Several months passed and the postings and artwork crossed every known line that a parent would tolerate as acceptable. Profanity was replete within her postings and she boasted on line about how her father permitted her and her brother to swear. She compared on-line the limits I set in our household to the care-free, lack of accountability that was the apparent way of life at her father's.

To my dismay, I learned that her father permitted my children to attend co-ed slumber parties with other teenagers whom I did not consider good influences to either of my children. How did I know these teenagers? Although I had never met most of them, I learned that they were peers at my children's school and they too, were posting things on the internet, which I also now spent time following because they posted back and forth to one another.

There seemed to be very little I could do as I watched my daughter's depression, behavior, and lack of respect for both myself and other adults in her life, go down the drain.

She began to do what she dubbed as "research" on the Columbine shootings. Her images of samurai-style slaughter began to focus on other individuals beside herself. Suddenly she was driven to prove to the world that she had something impor-tant to say, and that she wanted to go down in a "blaze of glory" and then be remembered for her profound statements and destructive actions.

She adopted a fascination with long black trench coats. She desperately had wanted one, and her reasons unbeknownst to me, she had talked me into allowing her to get one for her birthday. But now that I could see the connection between her coat and her postings, I was livid that I had unwittingly participated in her fantasy.

In addition, she was now making veiled and sometimes not so veiled threats against teachers and students. She openly discussed different ways of killing people and also herself. I saw one forum where she had openly asked the question, "how many of you seriously want to shoot up your school", (as if she was fishing for takers), to which varied replies were posted, ranging from "love to do it", to "sad to see you think that way." Even her peers were making comments about her postings, saying they were concerned for her negative and suicidal thoughts.

She seemed to deify Dylan Klebold and Eric Harris, the tragic youths who took thirteen lives and injured so many at Columbine High School in Littleton, Colorado on April 20, 1999.

She posted her writing assignments, and then regaled how her high school creative writing teacher had pulled her aside and questioned her about her poems that she had submitted for a grade. In them, she was very descriptive about the world around her, and her preoccupation with death and destruction was clearly evident. I read on-line that she had mocked the teacher's concern about them saying, "I laughed to myself and told her it was only a story."

Then my daughter criticized the teacher for being alert and trying to do her job. Still, the teacher never made any effort to contact either my ex nor myself with her concerns about our child's assignments, despite my having made it quite clear to the school that they should be watchfully alert for anything unusual coming from our child.

My child criticized authority, and she made comments saying she would love to "play with psychologists' minds" by telling them she "liked blood". She said she'd like to "go out in a blaze of glory", a "Mishima or a Columbine times ten."

Her postings were not at all average or what you'd expect from a girl who is a straight-A student. In fact, the symptoms of my child's depression acted out upon the internet and within her school assignments, convinced me that a child who I once thought would never do anything remotely violent, actually had the potential to harm herself or others. Since the time she had gone to live with her father, she had become almost unrecognizable to me in her behavior.

In fact, I would later learn that the events that preceeded the Columbine shootings were remarkably similar in tone to what I had discovered about my own daughter, but at the time she was posting, I knew very little about the events preceeding that famous incident.

[14]Dylan Klebold had, just weeks before the shootings, turned in a paper depicting tremendous violence. He had written, much like my daughter, a story about a trench-coat wearing warrior who killed students and detonated bombs. The creative writing teacher had also remarked her concerns about Dylan's writing, but unlike my daughter's teacher, had done more than just talk about the work, she had alerted his parents to his writings. And like my daughter, he had claimed it was "just a story."

Here I sat, with my own daughter copy-catting one of the worst incidents in recent history, and sick as I was, I did everything that I could think of, to bring the matter to people's attention. In retrospect, I probably could have tried other things, but I felt like I was walking on a tight rope and I couldn't think of any other options, and the people around us had no idea how to handle the situation.

On the one hand, I felt like I had to tread carefully because if my daughter discovered the extent of my knowledge of her activities, she might now go underground and I would have no ability to monitor what she was planning, if she was indeed planning anything, at all. Then again, if I exposed her in the wrong manner, I knew that the postings could land her in some serious hot water, and I did not want to jeopardize her academic future due to some bad judgements or serious depression on her part, whatever the case might be.

To make matters worse, about a week before the Red Lake, Minnesota school shooting, my daughter posted on-line a cartoon caracature of herself, shooting up the school. She was dressed as a samurai with a sword and dagger, in a long black trench coat. She had two machine guns, one in each hand, and there was blood and bodies strewn everywhere. Her talented depictions made the work all the more shocking, and she titled the picture, "Paint the School Red."

I felt a cold chill when I saw that piece of artwork. I had been following the sites she was visiting, and noticed the repeating theme of guns, suicide, violence and death everywhere. She was preoccupied with death and destruction and she openly talked about wanting to be glorified in a violent manner, dying at the end, as some sort of profound political statement about the misunderstood youth in our country.

When I came across that picture, I knew I would have to do something. She seemed to be teetering on the edge of a precipice and I desperately did not want her to fall. I had already contacted my sister-in-law in California, who had a psychology degree and who was a social worker. I had asked her for her opinion about what my daughter was posting, a month before I saw that picture.

Although I had not agreed with her, my sister-in-law had told me that it was not outside the realm of the unusual to see postings like some of what my daughter had written. However, even she was dismayed when she saw the latest image.

When I discovered a posting where my daughter was saying "goodbye" to her friends, I knew in my heart that she was planning to do something, and that *that* something might even include killing herself, if not others. Although I did not want to believe she was capable of that, her postings, her poetry, her illustrations and her confusing signals were no longer something I was willing to simply ignore. I could not live with the results if I chose to do nothing and she decided to do something stupid.

My husband and I went to our local sheriff's department and talked at length to them about the situation. It was Easter weekend in April of 2005, and just before the anniversary of the Columbine shootings. Due to some postings I had read, I was concerned that my daughter might be planning "something" to coincide with that date.

The police were a bit concerned but since my daughter lived with my ex, she was not within their jurisdiction. They dismissed us and told us to contact the police department in her home town and speak with them. I next tried to call my ex and tell him about my concerns, but all I got was his answering machine. I left a brief message that it was urgent that he call me. He did not return my call, and his lack of involvement and communication was exactly what I had expected from him.

We did contact the police in my ex's town, but they did not want anything to do with our situation. I felt like they did not take me seriously at all. They told me to contact the police liaison officer at the high school and speak with him. Since it was the weekend, I had to wait until Monday. We crossed our fingers that my daughter wouldn't do anything foolish all weekend.

On Monday, I called the school and was told that the officer was out on a hunting trip, and would not return until the following day. I sent him an email outlining what I had found and even sent him some internet links that were clear enough so that he could see for himself that what I was saying was true.

When he returned, we had a lengthy phone discussion and I asked him how he was planning to handle the situation. For one thing, she had posted some of her work, using the school's computers, and during school hours. For another, her father needed to be notified of what she was doing, especially as the majority of the activity was occurring from the computer at his home. I stressed the importance that the matter be handled delicately, as I knew that if her artwork was exposed in the wrong manner, that the media would probably have a field day with her.

She could already have been arrested and convicted of a misdemeanor or a felony if her threats had been taken seriously by someone. Anyone could have discovered her artwork at any time, as it was on a public forum, and they could have turned her in. I did not want that to happen to her, but I was aware of the seriousness of her work and wanted desperately for her to get counseling.

The police liaison officer assured me that he would only remove her from her classroom and have her speak with her guidance counselor. I agreed his idea would be acceptable. I would have to deal with the situation with my ex after that, but at least her internet activity would be noticed in a relatively safe manner, and she could finally obtain counseling—or so the officer led me to believe, anyway.

The rest of what happened next I discovered about a week later, as told to me by the school administrator during her post-incident pre-expulsion meeting.

From what I was told, the police liaison officer, the principal and possibly one of her teachers, performed a locker search on her. They had placed her personal items into bio-hazard baggies (which she saved and later thumb-tacked to her bedroom door at her father's house in a sign of defiance), and then they removed her from her classroom on an emergency detention.

They had found in her locker, notes indicating Columbine-type references, glorifications on her school schedule depicting violent holidays she would like to see, and including the names of various killers and pathological parties who were made famous in history. She had rewritten the school theme song á la Columbine, and they also found a map with what they deemed were exit points indicated. Whatever else they found had supported my concerns, and they apparently panicked.

The next thing I knew I was receiving a phone call from a social worker who kindly informed me that my child was being "processed" at the local hospital, and that she would then be transported via ambulance and straight jacket, to West Allis, to a mental health facility for a 72-hour observation period. (Interestingly, this was the same town where we had our previous home when the social worker accused us of living in a "changing urban environment". I found it a bit ironic that it was the exact place to which my child was sent by Walworth county social services. It was apparently a good enough town to treat my daughter for three days, but not good enough for her to live in permanently.)

When I was informed of my daughter's whereabouts, I think I said something like "Oh God", but all I could think of was my poor child and the fact that she was being taken to a mental hospital. That was not at *all* what I had been told was going to happen to her. In fact I had no idea just what an emergency detention *was*, and I had to have it explained to me by the social worker.

Once I realized the ramifications of all that was happening, my first thought was that my daughter was going to be very frightened. No matter what her mental state, she was still a child and this was not something any mother would have wished for her child, in any way shape or form. Had I known the consequences of my telling the authorities about her postings, I might have tried some other way to communicate, but I was very ill then, and had already exhausted what I thought were all valid attempts to communicate the situation while still protecting my daughter's future from overreactive authorities.

I knew that I had a tough choice to make, and despite not wanting to make that choice, I had done so out of love. I made what I felt was the best decision under the circumstances, with the knowledge that I had, and from my point of view, after I had exhausted everything else. Teenagers often put warning signs out there for their families to notice and yet the signs often go unheeded, with disastrous results. I did not want my daughter to be yet another statistic on the evening news.

The choice to report my daughter to school was not one that I took lightly but it was one that I could live with. It was far better to me to be held up on a stick for turning her in than to perhaps run the risk of losing her from suicide or worse.

I just had no idea that the school officials would react in the manner in which they had. But the Minnesota shooting had just happened *that same week*, and teenagers were being arrested all over the country for perceived verbal threats that were not even as blatant or graphic as the ones my daughter had posted. She was very lucky I had turned her in, because the consequences of her actions could have been a whole lot worse had she been discovered by anyone else.

At the hospital, she was diagnosed as clinically depressed and placed on suicide watch. During the meeting with the psychologist, I was told that if she exhibited her depression for a long period of time, that she should probably be on anti-depressants. I disagreed with the doctor, and said there was no way I would allow her to be on those, as I felt her problems to be situational in nature, or at least that if there could be something medically wrong with her, she did not need to be medicated before she was even diagnosed.

As you can expect, once my ex-husband was informed of the incident, he took it upon himself to immediately discredit me in whatever manner he possibly could. He went to great lengths to at first deny his insurance information to the intake coordinator, leaving them to contact me and ask if I would be the responsible party. I told them that by law and court decree he was to provide the insurance for the children and I provided them with his insurance information, for our daughter's benefit.

Additionally, he must have given the psychologist one heck of a story about me, because she quickly dismissed both my concerns and me physically from the parental meeting. I was not even told what the procedures were, and the psychologist immediately deferred all my questions to my ex-husband. "Oh, its being handled," was what she kept repeating to me when I inquired about my daughter's welfare. How was she getting home? When was she being released? Did she have enough clothing (I had brought her some, because my ex hadn't even thought that she had nothing with her for the three-day stint).

The psychologist ushered me and my husband out the door like we were unwanted guests. The details for her stay and release were completely handled between the psychologist and my ex. Correspondence sent to the psychologist after the fact in the form of letters and emails were never replied to. Phone calls were never returned when I left them. I was being completely ignored and I could not for the life of me, figure out why.

The psychologist *had* questioned me about *my* personal background and her assistant had carefully taken notes of everything I said, especially things that were of a personal nature. Some of the questions they asked me were absolutely unessential in evaluating my child's behavior.

I noticed this offensive behavior and commented a bit sarcastically because the assistant and another gal were whispering to each other about me and in front of me. I said, "make sure you write that one down" when I answered one of their obnoxious questions that had nothing to do with our situation. I felt curiously like *I* was the one being evaluated for mental illness.

The lack of respect afforded to me went further. When I made a comment about how I had no knowledge of my child being ED'd out of school, the psychologist said "at that point, the school can do that, they don't have to ask all the mommies and the daddies for their permission", she condescendingly told me. What a jerk I thought to myself, and this is supposed to be a doctor–a PhD?

A few weeks later when I obtained records about my daughter's stay at the facility, I quickly learned why I had been treated so harshly. My ex-husband had carefully made allegations to the staff that I suffered from mental illness. He made claims about my "doing this" (meaning sending my child to a psych ward), in order to "bankrupt" him and to "teach our daughter a lesson".

The staff had noted "mother may have mental problems" in one area along with my ex's claims that were carefully recorded. In another area, notations were present that again underscored that I actually *had* mental problems. And I had never exhibited anything of the sort, nor had I been diagnosed. It was all an attempt to discredit me by my ex, and he had been very successful. If I had had any money at all, I would have filed a slander suit against him faster than you can say slander suit. Now his intense desire to ruin my life was stepped up another notch and he was using our daughter's unfortunate situation to do so.

The good part about my daughter's behaviors being discovered, was that she became aware of the fact that someone *was* watching her. A child that clearly had been crying out for someone to notice her, had after all, been seen by me.

My crime at being a loving parent resulted in my being heavily chastized by my daughter, who went back on-line at her father's house and proceeded to ream me out publicly for "my" behavior.

She was blaming me for being sent to the psychiatric hospital when I hadn't even known it would be a possibility. Of course, my actions led to that decision by the school, but ultimately the responsibility for the event should fall squarely upon her shoulders, as she was the one who did the posting, and who possessed the things found within her locker, not I.

Naturally her peers said extremely unkind things about me on-line. A very graphic, very painful torture leading to my death was clearly described multiple times. The juvenile admonishment did not bother me so much as the fact that she was still on-line and posting away, both at her father's home and at school.

Because of accusations my ex had made about me to the school staff, my credibility was destroyed. Neither the conversations I had with the school administrator nor the principal nor teachers fell on receptive ears. Later on, phone calls, emails and letters to the staff also failed to elicit very much of a response from them. Again, I was ignored–presumably because of what my ex had already told these people. It certainly wasn't because I had approached them in any negative fashion. I was a parent with a legitimate concern and I made every effort to be as composed and helpful as possible. After the principal wrote me off by saying "I'll check into it and get back to you," that was the last I heard from him, even after I left three phone messages requesting a call-back.

During our only meeting, despite my asking the school to block the internet site that my child and her fellow students were utilizing during class time, they ignored me, claiming it was not their responsibility. "You just had a student you ED'd out of school–when *will* it be your responsibility?" I implored. And yet for a full fifteen months after the incident, my child and others like her posted happily away, during school hours, using school computers. It was not until I could convince her new counselor, the following year of my concerns that the high school *finally* blocked the internet site that the students were abusing on school time and in an unhealthy manner.

My daughter's father did nothing about her computer use at home either. Finally after a few months he apparently had attempted to temporarily ground her from using the computer, because her brother told me of this. But in short, she found ways to work around her father's knowledge of her computer use, and back on-line she would go. Eventually he did not bother to monitor her usage at all, and she was free to resume her internet activities, much to my dismay. Next she posted a horrific image of a child who had just been released from an institution. The image showed a girl smiling wickedly, with the smile held forcibly open by huge safety pins pinned to her skin, which pulled her mouth upward. Blood was trickling down the face, and there was a gaping, open wound on the top of the person's head into which a hypodermic needle was placed and injecting "proper" thoughts into her head.

There were comments like "see, we made her smile" and things of that nature. She was mocking the system, making fun of the people who had detained and evaluated her; and quite literally the entire process.

In my opinion, at this point, she had learned absolutely nothing from the experience except what I had expected her to do; which was to make an effort to become less noticeable. She did this by changing her moniker or handle on the internet. Within a short time, I once again discovered her activities by being a bit sleuthy and watching what her friends were posting.

And of course, since Lyme disease had never even been a question in the grand scheme of these activities, it remained completely unrecognized as a possible causative factor for all of her depressed and bad behaviors, so her freedom to act up and carry on, continued wholly unabated.   ❖

❖ Chapter 10 ❖

Right All Along

During my daughter's escapades, I was in the worst stages of my Lyme symptoms in years. I had been unable to eat normally for the better part of two years. The nutritional deficiencies brought with them a host of symptoms, especially fatigue, but my Lyme was at a point where a diagnosis was absolutely critical. I had been on a long downward slope in my health and I was getting much sicker.

Even during the psych evaluation of my daughter, I had just completed yet another abdominal surgery, this time for another growth on my remaining ovary. I was barely a week out of the hospital when I had to deal with my daughter's problems. I also had no real use of my left arm and hand, could no longer walk unsupported, could not drive, and had great difficulty with daily function.

I had to have help with basic things like putting a sweater over my head because I wasn't strong enough or had enough range of motion to dress myself properly.

I had to have my husband help me with anything and everything I tried to do. Becoming completely dependent upon another human being was not something I took lightly by any means. I had been independent all my life and this was extremely difficult for me. He was now cooking all my meals, doing all the shopping, driving, chores, dealing with our pets, kids, phone calls, and supporting us while I lay around unable to participate in the simplest of activities.

I had all the major physical and neurological symptoms of Lyme disease and I can honestly say that I had been sick for many years, but now my body was rapidly failing me. I was declining physically, emotionally and cognitively. I couldn't remember what I was doing or where I was going. I felt confused and the brain fog made concentration impossible.

All that my children ever heard was "mom is sick" and they basically ignored me most of the time because I could not participate in anything they were doing. I could often be found in bed during their weekends or lying about on the sofa; and they began to resent me and my supposed illness. They made subtle comments about my not really being sick, especially during my anaphylactic reactions, and I remember being the butt of many a joke. Although they were scolded for their unkind remarks, I knew that the words they repeated had originated from one source, and that source was probably their father, who had openly mocked my illness in court many times.

Every so often on a good day, I was lucky enough to find time and the ability to read, and I came across the alternative practice of NAET. For those who do not know what this is, it is the elimination of allergies using a technique invented by Dr. Devi Nambudripad M.D. (WI), D.C., L.Ac., Ph.D. (Acu.). Since I had so many of what I believed to be allergies to foods and chemicals, I thought I had nothing to lose and everything to gain by pursuing this alternative medicine.

I did not know much about it at the time, but I thought if there was anything I could do to discover what was wrong with me physically, then I would try absolutely anything that made sense to me. I had already tried antibiotics, herbs, essential oils, accupuncture, traditional doctors, deep tissue massage, multiple surgeries, prayer groups, magnetic therapy and a few things I cannot for the life of me figure out why I tried them. Knowing I had nothing to lose except my illness, I thought what the heck, and decided to give NAET a try.

My practitioner was a registered nurse, and someone who also worked at a hospice. In her "spare" time, she was a certified NAET/ NMT practitioner and although she was 18 miles from my home, I decided I needed to force myself to drive there once a week for a month, to see if this avenue would prove fruitful.

I found the process interesting, valid and even helpful, but more importantly, one afternoon she casually mentioned a seminar that she had recently attended. A doctor there had discussed treating his Lyme disease patients with nutritional supplements. "Hey," I remember saying as I sat upright on the folding table. "Can you tell me who that was? I have sworn all these years that I have had Lyme, but I have never been able to get anybody to listen to me." She provided me with the man's name, though she regretfully could not remember where he had his practice, only that it was located somewhere within our state.

Undaunted by this fact, I telephoned many medical facilities that afternoon and I did not let the sun set before I tracked down the doctor and his treatment facility, which was located (lucky for me), only about an hour away from our home.

I met for several hours with this very caring, very thorough, physician. He was provided with copious amounts of my medical records which he carefully studied. I described to him as much as I could remember about all the tests, procedures and medications I had taken over the course of the last twelve-and-a-half years. I shared my suspicions that I had Lyme disease with him and relayed how my doctors had ignored my many requests to be tested properly and treated for Lyme.

Then he shared with me his diagnostic hypothesis, which he said might be confirmed by blood tests which he would also perform. He said that after carefully reviewing my extensive medical history, that there was no doubt in his mind whatsoever that I did indeed, probably have Lyme disease. He said in his opinion, my former doctors should have noticed my illness somewhere along the line, because my laboratory tests over the years clearly showed a persistent disease state.

He told me the lab facility that he used was "pretty good" at detecting Lyme and said that we would know for certain in a couple of weeks, one way or the other about the Lyme diagnosis.

I remember thinking "I *knew* it!" and felt a little bit elated because finally someone had validated my suspicions. When I left his office, I was so happy at finally being diagnosed that I began to cry. But I was then so unhappy that I *was* finally diagnosed, that I cried even more.

It had taken twelve-and-a-half years for me to get the diagnosis that I had suspected at the very onset of my illness, and I could not understand why it had taken so darned long for someone to finally listen to me. Because of that, I felt cheated out of over a decade of my life, and now carried the uncertainty of my ability to recover the health that I had once freely enjoyed.

In time, test results in the form of a CDC positive IgM and an equivocal (by CDC standards) IgG Western Blot combined with my clinical history and known exposure to a tick bite confirmed the Lyme diagnosis. In addition, I learned that I had a number of co-infections as well, so those had to be treated in addition to the Lyme disease.

As it turned out, at the time of my diagnosis, my doctor was better at diagnosing Lyme disease than he was at knowing precisely how to treat it (not his fault). He was the first to admit that he did not know enough about Lyme yet to actually cure it, but he was at least willing to try different treatment options with me.

In frustration during one appointment, I did lose patience with him when he openly stated that "antibiotics don't work on Lyme patients." While I liked him much as a physician, I took his statement as a sign that perhaps I should search elsewhere for a more Lyme-literate doctor for my acute treatment and perhaps return to him when he had learned a little bit more about the disease.

I was worried about what kind of treatment I would receive, but my fears were probably more due to my own lack of knowledge about treating this disease than anything. I attempted to get my hands on any book I could find about Lyme and read up on the subject as much as I could. I spent hours on the internet trying to find information about the illness, and its treatment.

The information that I found was helpful but often conflicting and confusing. There seemed to be two camps of thought. One group had many doctors believing that Lyme disease is easily curable with a short course of antibiotics, say 28 or 30 days in duration. Apparently all of my previous doctors had been members of this "camp".

I knew that I had received many doses of different medications over the years, and here I was, in the throws of Lyme disease, and faring far worse than what the doctors were claiming I should be. According to them, I should have been long-since cured of Lyme.

I could tell from my symptoms that I had never been cured of Lyme disease. Ever since that day way back in 1992 when I had my initial flu symptoms, I never again felt well, and I mean not one single day went by *ever* that I can honestly say that I felt completely well.

The feeling of the presence of the Lyme spirochete in my body was a constant companion, one with which I was all too familiar. If I had been cured, that feeling should have gone away, but here I was a dozen years later and Lyme was still persistently affecting me in every possible manner and I was very ill.

Actually what I had, I found out is referred to as Chronic Lyme Neuroborreliosis, a bunch of big words to describe a really serious illness. I did not feel like my body had some auto-immune process happening, as one doctor had hypothesized. The stabbing, shooting pains that felt like I was being eaten alive inside told me that the spirochete was now extremely active in my system.

I decided to go along with the doctors in the "other" camp who said that Lyme disease could and should be treated with antibiotics, perhaps even intravenous antibiotics, and for lengthy time periods. Serious disease, I rationalized, required serious measures. I was about as seriously ill as I ever cared to be, and had been, for many years.

In time, my diagnosis of Lyme disease was leaked through my children to my ex-husband, and he wasted no time in attempting to bring this issue to light in the court of law. He managed to drag us back to court on an unrelated matter, and interject the "necessity" for him and his attorney to dumpster-dive through my private medical files in order to "prove" that I did not have Lyme disease, as I was suddenly now claiming, as it affected my ability to pay him child support.

For a reason that escapes me now, the courts agreed with them, and allowed them to subpoena my records and force me to sign release forms to enable them to facilitate this process. It is incredibly embarrassing to have your ex and his attorney (or anybody else for that matter), plow through what are supposed to be confidential medical records for no good reason. I felt violated once again and it made me very angry that the court was allowing them to do this; and for what purpose, I was yet unclear.

I did my best attempt at blocking the process while still complying with the court order. I granted them one-time access *only* to tests that could confirm the diagnosis of Lyme disease, and nothing more, which properly frustrated them for the time being. I felt strongly that they had no business digging around in my medical files, not that there was anything there that I needed to be ashamed of, or protective of, other than my right to privacy; and I felt very strongly about that issue.

During this process, my new Lyme physician was harrassed by both my medical records situation and also my ex and his attorney's attempts to have him testify against me in the trial. He reluctantly declined to treat me, citing that he didn't get involved in court matters. Because of my ex and his attorney, I in effect, lost the only doctor that I knew of at the time, who was willing and able to treat my condition.

This was infuriating as you can well imagine, because it had taken so long for me just to obtain a diagnosis; and my ex-husband and his attorney's interference was now blocking both my ability and my right to become well. Nevertheless I persevered in my search for another Lyme literate doctor within our state.

I did happen to locate a physician, one of only three that I have found to date in Wisconsin, who was willing to treat my Lyme disease with a course of intravenous antibiotics. He performed more tests than my initial Lyme doctor had, and after examining me, told me that I was probably going to require immediate IV treatment for my symptoms.

First the doctor wanted to perform an MRI on my brain to check for lesions, because I had so many symptoms of multiple sclerosis. I had been diagnosed with possible MS in the past by neurologists, but all they did was prescribe amyltriptilene, which is an anti-depressant designed to basically be a bandaid for my symptoms, and that was not good enough for me. I did not take either their prescription nor their diagnosis seriously. I had some-how instinctively known that I did not have MS, though I agreed that some of the symptoms were remarkably similar in nature.

I agreed to do the brain scan, but during the first MRI my little Lyme critters kept causing me to have panic attacks. I had to reschedule the MRI and do it on a different date, which was both embarrassing and frustrating. My doctor prescribed valium for me to take, but in the end I toughed it out and fought with myself to remain both calm and relaxed rather than have to take unnec-essary drugs. After all, I had many MRI's before and had never experienced this problem with them. After reviewing the report from the MRI, it was determined that I had lesions on my brain and that the eight week IV treatment should begin immediately.

I was to have my husband drive me to the hospital and have the infusions done there due to my "weird" allergic reactions. It was a frightening prospect for me to have a picc line inserted. (A picc line is a peripherally inserted central catheter, which is a tube that commonly runs from the inside of your upper arm, into your chest with the tip resting in a large vein just above your heart). But having a picc line was a small price to pay as far as I was concerned, in order to finally be on the road to some level of physical wellness, especially after all the years of being ill.

I desperately wanted to see if the drugs would alleviate my symptoms, especially my pain, clarity of thought, my balance and coordination problems and my inability to use my left arm and hand.

The doctor prescribed zoloft and benadryl because my body reacted to the saline flush used to clean out the central catheter. I tried to tell him that the saline had preservatives in it and that they were directly responsible for the allergic reactions, but he insisted that he knew better and deemed my reactions simple panic attacks.

My husband and I tried to explain that if the nurse used dextrose instead of saline, that the problem would not recur and he quickly took offense at us trying to "tell him" how to treat me.

We talked as nicely as we could but this doctor who was already in his eighties, was extremely arrogant. He insisted that we knew nothing about medicine and that he was the doctor and that we should listen to him. He actually said to me, "you're just the patient, what do you know?" Only after he actually witnessed one of my severe reactions first-hand did he relent and prescribed dextrose instead of the saline. But from that moment on, he had a very bad attitude where I was concerned.

All we were trying to do was alert him to known problems with the saline flush, and he thought we were trying to tell him how to practice medicine, so we quickly had problems communicating with this closed-minded physician.

Nevertheless, we persevered each day and my husband changed his work schedule and worked half-days so that we could travel the hundred or so mile round trip each day. Most of the time, the infusions went well, but when they did not, I was in for a rough drive home with nausea and other symptoms with which to deal while my hubby drove frantically home, trying to beat the clock before I needed to use the bathroom.

After a week of this, it was determined that I could do the infusions at home, and home care was ordered. It was not without its problems however, as I quickly discovered. The home care nurses had no intention of seeing me more than twice to teach me how to self-infuse, and then they would only appear once per week, and only to perform routine checks on my blood pressure.

The thought of self-administered IV medications scared me because I had never done anything like that before in my life, and I really did not feel physically up to handling the situation.

Making matters worse, my husband had missed so much time off work just in the one week of driving to the hospital that he was now backlogged and couldn't seem to catch up. He had to work overtime to correct this, and it was a good thing the work was available, because the cost of the medication that was not covered by insurance was staggering. The IV medicines alone cost us several thousand dollars every week and I was going to require at least eight weeks of them. Then there were the doctor fees, the hospital, the other antibiotics, drug supplies and nursing care to pay for.

In the end, I only ever received two weeks of IV therapy. I suffered severe Jarich-Herxheimer reactions, (a complex allergic response to antigens released from the dying spirochetes), to the infusions daily and those were rough enough all by themselves. The drugs were incredibly hard on my system, and being little more than a hundred pounds, the doseage levels were exceedingly high for me and my body quickly had problems with them.

My husband and I asked the doctor if he would please adjust my dosage as I was literally passing out each and every day immediately following my infusions. I would black out for an hour and a half or two full hours. I would then wake up later with the IV still attached to the IV pump, waiting for me to unhook myself.

In addition, I had intense pain over my liver (remember I had no gallbladder); my skin turned a ghastly yellow hue, and I was unbearably short of breath. I had terrible chest pain and got immediately sick following each infusion.

Pulsing the doses helped but as soon as they resumed, by the time the third gram of Rocephin entered my bloodstream and mixed with the other medications, I would grow nauseated and dizzy and black out again or have to go immediately to the bathroom with horrible diarrhea. I lost twelve pounds in two weeks.

As I had always done, I begged the doctor to listen to me, but he flatly refused. My husband and I told the doctor repeatedly of our concern about the high drug dosage. His argument was that he had given one of his male patients six grams of IV Rocephin per day for six months and *that* patient had done just fine. His arrogance was perplexing—I wasn't *that patient*, he probably weighed much more than I, and furthermore, I wasn't even male.

The medication was not treating me well at all, and was adding to my already overtaxed system. I knew how inordinately ill I was now becoming, and it was outside the realm of what could be expected from typical treatments. Instead of listening or understanding however, the doctor instead coldly told me "grit your teeth and get through it." He laughed at my complaints of "aches and pains" despite my attempts to tell him that the aches and pains he mentioned were *not* in fact what I was complaining about.

I did grit my teeth, a lot, and yet I knew with every fiber of my being that if I continued in the same manner as I was going, that the cumulative effects of all the medications were going to be, quite literally, the death of me, and I honestly did not want to die. I had the feeling like I had so many times in my life when *you just know* that something isn't right, and my treatments weren't right—not by a long shot.

I knew that I could tolerate nearly all the infusion, but as soon as the levels got past a certain point, there was just too much medication. I guess you could compare it to being really drunk. I don't drink but did a few times when I was in my early twenties. When you drink, you can have a drink or two and be tipsy. That is very different from being drunk. When I received any amount under a certain dose of the medications, I was fine and went about my day herxing along. But the minute the dosage was exceeded beyond a certain point, all hell would break loose. That is how I could tell that my dose was too strong.

I learned long ago to trust my gut feeling, and my guts were telling me that something was very wrong with the amount of medication I was receiving for my body weight. This was not just the effects of dying spirochetes nor the combination of medications. It was directly caused by the *amount* I was being given and I could actually feel it harming me with every infusion.

After my husband and I had our final (and heated on the doctor's part) conversation about my situation, our doctor said that he no longer wanted to treat me. He claimed that we were trying to tell him how to administer medicine, and we defended ourselves from his claims. The doctor had *himself* told us that if we had *any problems* with the at-home treatments that he was to be notified at once. Then when my husband *did* call him to tell him that I was passing out from the drugs, the doctor refused to take any of his calls.

We begged the doctor to please reconsider his position, because I needed treatment. In the end he said he would "think about it" and that he'd call us in another week after he "rested" and decided what he was going to do with "difficult" me.

We were supposed to blindly accept the problems that my body was having with the medication because you don't dare question your doctor about the *very effects* of which he had told us to be mindful. At the beginning of the program, my husband had asked "what kind of things should we watch out for?" The doctor had replied, "well, if she passes out or anything like that, call me." Here I had been *doing* just that (passing out), and yet when we tried to tell him, he didn't want to deal with the problem and instead tried to say that we were *telling him what to do*, which did not make any sense at all.

I don't know about you, but in our opinion this was not the ideal doctor-patient relationship as he certainly did not seem to care very much about his patient. In the end, he never did call us back, and I was left sitting at home without medication, and with inter-rupted treatments. Home alone and unable to flush my own picc line myself because I only had one hand and no extension line, I had to contact the pharmaceutical company and wait for them to deliver the needed supplies, because the doctor left me without treatment and I needed to maintain my equipment or risk infec-tion. This was infuriating, not to mention completely unethical.

Not to prove a point, but I began to get better as soon as the infusions ended. I still had to deal with the after-effects of the medications, the Lyme and the herxheimer reactions, but the sickening feeling I got with each "overdosed" infusion miracu-lously disappeared.

I tried to see the only other doctor I could find who might be able to continue my treatments, but he refused to use the existing picc line because of "legal ramifications". In other words, since he hadn't ordered the existing picc line to be inserted, he was not about to utilize it. If I wanted him to treat me, I would have to have *another* picc line inserted, by him, and this one pulled.

The central catheter had been inside of my body for four weeks now, and the line was beginning to show signs of infection. Because the original doctor would not answer his phone mes-sages, I could not get him to order that the line be pulled. I had already experienced septicemia once in my life, and I well knew the dangers of having an open wound offering a free ride for bacteria to my bloodstream. I then telephoned the interventional radiologist at the hospital who had been responsible for inserting the line, and explained my predicament. With just one phone call, he made the original doctor order it be removed.

He said that he was very upset at my doctor's behavior, and suggested that I report him to the hospital administrator at once. I did want to do that, but declined to do so only because if he was indeed helping other patients, that our misunderstanding, if you wanted to call it that, should perhaps be overlooked.

Not to sound grandiose, but just in case our doctor was held accountable for leaving me hanging there without treatment and an infected picc line for no reason we could ascertain, perhaps our complaints would lead to discipline of some kind, preventing him from treating other patients. We did not want to be the cause of that in the off-chance it happened, because we knew how difficult it was just to get *any* kind of treatment for Lyme disease, even ill-treatment.

I have since learned from other Lyme patients that this doctor had different issues with them, and that he was difficult with everyone, so it was not just me and my husband who were having problems with him. Perhaps he was, in his eighties, well past his retirement age. Perhaps his skills, although valuable, were better off passed on to someone younger. In the end, we learned that he was no longer taking new patients but that his son was taking over his practice, so maybe he *was* at the end of his serviceable medical career.

I was now aware of the political controversy surrounding Lyme disease, but I did not know enough about the treatments or their dosages to know if what my doctor had done was correct or not, and I did not want to be the judge of that, so in the end we figured we'd leave well enough alone.

After the IV treatments, and with my picc line finally pulled, I spent the next six months recovering from the ordeal I had just been through. My body had a tough time with this process and I spent hours in the sun trying to convert my yellow skin tones back to either a toasty brown or at least my pasty-white normal hue.

In the beginning, I could only lay in bed or on the couch. Walking any distance at all, even a few feet, was virtually impossible. I was inordinately weak and not at all well. But in time and with perseverance, I managed to build up enough strength so that I could walk a bit around the yard.

When the next door neighbors saw me laying in the hammock at the end of the summer, they jokingly commented on my "easy life" without knowing what I had just been through or that I was desperately ill. We had not lived in our house very long before I began treatment for Lyme disease, so no one really knew our situation, except for my neighbors across the street, who helpfully babysat our pets during our daily hospital visits.

Despite the difficulties I had with the medications, the herxheimer reactions and the too-high levels of antibiotics in my system, by October, six months after beginning IV treatments, the paralysis in my arm finally dissipated. Over the next six months, the majority of my neurological symptoms would fall by the wayside, especially the more severe ones.

While I still had a laundry list of symptoms with which to deal, I began to function again. Gone was much of the mental dullness and brain fog I experienced, along with the confusion and poor memory problems. I felt a bit like myself again, and I welcomed any progress, no matter how small. Slowly but surely, as each day progressed, I found my strength returning and the ability to do more things a welcome change from the life that I had been living for so long.

In time, I could drive again. While I could not drive for very long or at very fast speeds (because I could not seem to process movement in space properly); I *could* drive slowly around town. So venturing out to get the mail from the post office four blocks away became a really big deal for me.

I felt so blessed when I could finally walk around our yard without being exhausted and needing a nap. I thanked God when I could make it through a single afternoon without needing to lie down and rest. When my sleep disturbances improved, I was so very grateful the first time I slept through an entire night–the first time I had done so, in years. I smiled as I noticed new hairs beginning to return to the top of my head.

As I got better and my knowledge about Lyme disease grew, I began to think about all the illnesses and symptoms my children had endured over the years. I reflected on my daughter's diagnosis of depression and my son's behavioral problems, when all of a sudden the thought occurred to me to test my children for Lyme disease.

They had both experienced weird rashes on their legs when they were small. I thought about all the illnesses they had when they were growing up, the incontinence, the infections, high fevers, and other things left unexplained by their doctors. Yes, I now wondered if both of my children had been exposed to Lyme disease at the same time that I had been, way back during that summer of 1992.

My daughter was still suffering from headaches, light sensitivity, ringing in her ears, stomach aches, menstrual problems, joint pains, suicidal/homicidal thoughts, behavioral problems and depression.

My son had also been complaining of light sensitivity, headaches, bone and joint problems, particularly in his knees and back; and was having major anger issues. His behavior was the pits at times, and practically anything would set him off. I saw patterns to his behavior that mirrored my own, and I gained a new understanding of what he was going through. I made the decision to have my children tested for Lyme disease.

Convincing a child to let you take him or her to the doctors to have blood drawn, if you are a parent, is sometimes far easier said than done. I was surprised that my daughter complied but my son would put up a fight. In the end, common sense overruled their objections and I made an appointment with my general practitioner, to talk to him about testing them both for Lyme disease.

I also had continued my research on the internet and in the library on Lyme disease. I was greatly dismayed to learn about the problems with diagnosis and treatment, and the sometime inaccuracy of the lab tests or their interpretation. But I felt certain that the laboratory that had correctly diagnosed me with Lyme disease should be trusted to test my children as well.

My wonderful GP, who admittedly knows little about Lyme disease but who is open to learning about it, agreed that both of the children's medical histories warranted at least a Western Blot for Lyme, and he ordered the blood to be drawn.

The lab tests returned a couple of weeks later and revealed that both of my children had also tested positive for Lyme disease. My daughter had tested positive by CDC standards, although my son's test had returned equivocal by CDC standards. Still there *was* Borrelia burgdorferi DNA found in his samples, just not enough to be considered positive according to the narrow criteria defined by the CDC. In mine and many people's opinions, (including prominent physicians), you can't have Bb present and *not* have been exposed to Lyme disease at some point.

The Lyme DNA simply does not magically appear all by itself nor does its presence, even in a small amount, mean that it does *not* exist just because someone set the criteria standard bar too low. To me that's a lot like finding cancer cells in someone's body but then attempting to deny one has cancer because there are only a few of them, despite whether or not that cancer is actively reproducing or in an undetectable, remissive state. Many Lyme patients are denied a diagnosis and essential treatment because they simply do not meet the criteria, which is often misinterpreted, and which desperately needs to be updated for any one of these patients to ever get well.

After reviewing the children's test results, our physician remarked that he was intensely interested in our family's case because of our recent lab results and long-standing history of symptoms. He even expressed interest in learning more about Lyme disease, and because I ran a support group, asked me to provide him with more information about it.

My doctor had never seen a family who still tested positive so many years after being exposed, and who were still experiencing symptoms after the "normal" 30-day treatment of doxycycline.

My guess is that he truly had not seen nor diagnosed many Lyme patients during his relatively short career (he was only in his early thirties). I applaud him for being open-minded enough to allow the testing to take place, and also to being willing to learn more about this devastating disease, even if he is a bit cautious about doing so. **If more physicians were willing to listen to their patients and step up to the plate when proven correct, Lyme disease could quickly become erradicated.**

The doctor prescribed his usual treatment for Lyme disease, and that which he was "allowed" to prescribe, which was thirty days of doxycycline. In my book, anything was going to be helpful to my children, even if the medication was only a short-term fix. If we could kill any spirochetes at all during that time period, perhaps I could buy my children some valuable time before we began another treatment regimen.

As I suspected, the children's father fought me on the whole idea of our children having Lyme disease. To make matters worse, my son was convinced by his father that he did not *have* Lyme disease, because his test was only equivocal by CDC standards, and not fully positive. Naturally, my children's father refused to allow them to take their medication while they were at his home. As it was now the summer months, my visitation allowed me to have them for an entire week at a time, with my ex having alternate weeks.

Over the course of two months, my children took their thirty-day supply of medication, one week at a time, with a complete week (their father's) as a resting period. What they were doing in effect was pulsing a dose of doxycycline every other week. Although it was not the ideal way to treat their symptoms, it was far better than doing nothing at all.

The effects of the doxy on their system was immediate and dramatic. For the first time in over a year, my daughter's depression seemed to lift quite a bit. My son stopped complaining about every ache and pain that he experienced and both of their attitudes improved dramatically. I was getting my children back on some level, and it was all because they had finally been correctly diagnosed–even if it was some thirteen years after first becoming ill.   ❖

❖ Chapter 11 ❖

Court of Fools

As if Lyme disease was not enough of a problem with which to deal, throughout the years 1997 through the present, I have had to continually deal with family and court problems. You have read about some of the surgeries that also got thrown into the mix; the real estate deal gone badly, and four separate moves into three different towns, two of them within eight months of each other. There are many other events that passed my way that are not included in the book, but I have detailed some of the most important items because I feel they are directly connected to Lyme disease.

Although the addage is "when it rains it pours", my life has provided me with a tsunami of events, lending a new meaning to that phrase. Despite this, I have continued to struggle to keep my head above water; sometimes dog-paddling just to stay afloat. The best way I have found to survive difficulty is to focus on one event at a time, and set a goal for yourself to get through it. As *Winston Churchill* has said, "When you're going through hell, keep going", and I did just that.

Lyme disease is a most difficult foe with which to do battle, and as if the devastating symptoms are not enough to handle, the ignorance surrounding the disease and the discrimination that abounds makes it doubly hard.

The most important thing that I lacked in my experience was a good support system. My family did not understand any of the aspects of Lyme disease, nor how it could change a person from a rational, functioning human being into a sad shell of their former self.

Family and friends turned away when my illness became inconvenient for them to understand, and as I became more unreliable for family functions. The public chastized me for utilizing a motorized cart in the grocery store or for parking in the handicapped zone when I could no longer walk far on my own, but could not get a doctor to complete the handicapped request form issued by the state department of motor vehicles for me so I could be legitimately registered as handicapped.

When my face was paralyzed, I stood humiliated and embarrassed at the looks on the faces of my co-workers, shopkeepers and others when I appeared in public. I was ridiculed by many people when my thinking became unclear, or when I could no longer do the simplest tasks, making others lose patience with me for my "stupidity".

I watched myself act out irrationally which led to my losing a good-paying job that I liked very much, because I had no control over the effects of Lyme disease on my brain and body.

I was accused by social workers of having a face "full of rage", and having "eyes of pain", which were mere echoes of the undiagnosed illness I carried inside of my body. And my doctors no longer paid any attention to me as I tried in vain to get someone to listen to my hypothesis that I had been exposed to Lyme disease.

When my ex-husband set out to destroy my credibility, he had an assistant, one of whom he was unaware, and whose name was Lyme disease. Because my symptoms affected me each and every day over the course of many years, I slowly deteriorated in bodily function, personality and clarity of thinking. He took advantage of my lack of control because of the illness preying upon my brain and body and parlayed it into something it was not, which was supposed mental illness.

My ex created a very long paper trail that spans the length of three or four years, and the family court has unwittingly assisted him in that process. If I had not been suffering from the effects of Lyme disease, I could have handled the process of him trying to remove my children from my life with a laugh and a resolve to not let the court or him get the better of us. However, because I was so ill with so many things happening simultaneously, I was completely at a loss as to how to cope with the changes that were being flung in my direction, one after the other.

As a result, I did not always conduct myself in the best manner possible, and the court officers could tell that *something* was going on, though they could not put their finger on exactly what that something actually was.

What the court-ordered counselors had seen was simply a physically and emotionally shattered woman who was very ill, and in fear of losing her children to a man who would create so many lies that he and everyone around him, actually believed them.

My insistence that I did not feel well at each counseling session reached deaf ears. "I don't feel well" does not adequately describe the symptoms of Lyme disease nor how one feels when recovering from abdominal surgery. But that was as articulate as I could be at the time, due to the effects of then unrecognized Lyme disease on my brain.

The children's guardian ad litem, who seemed a bit reluctant to do his job, declared in court that I had a full plate. He could see that there was something happening to me that was perhaps outside the realm of normal, but he too, could not determine exactly what it was he was seeing. Instead of doing their jobs and investigating further our situation, the court officers instead put forth the minimum required effort and made a judgement about our home situation without being clear on what they were seeing.

If any of them had actually performed a proper home evaluation or spoken to the over thirty-six personal references I had supplied them, they would have seen a starkly contrasting view of me through others' eyes. This should have led them to question why my behavior had appeared so out-of-the-ordinary during counseling. I was not suffering from emotional and mental problems, I was suffering from an undiagnosed infection in my body and brain.

The fact that I was so ill and continually declining in health also seemed to escape those present in the court room. The judges occasionally made comments about my ability to testify, while the opposition's attorneys made snide remarks about me and the illness that I had supposedly fabricated. At first they tried to argue that I was not really sick at all, but that I had *imagined* that I was ill in order to avoid paying child support to my ex-husband.

I faced contempt motions for this, and was found in contempt a couple of times, once narrowing missing a six-month stint in prison by paying over a thousand dollars to my ex-husband immediately. A second time I had to pay four hundred dollars to my ex's attorney for court costs for him "having" to bring the motion before the courts.

When I finally was diagnosed with Lyme disease in 2004, I received a temporary reprieve from the harrassment of my imaginary illness, at least on the stand. The court was reticent in accepting that Lyme disease could have "done so much" to me that it prevented me from working. My ex's attorney even declared that he knew several people who had multiple sclerosis and even *they* were still working. As if Lyme disease was as prevalent or as simple as the common cold.

Unfortunately, Lyme disease elicits no respect in a court of law, at least not yet. Lyme patients are ridiculed, prosecuted for their illness, and held accountable for behaviors for which they have no real control or awareness. I witnessed firsthand just how cruelly an illness can devastate a family when manipulated by persons who lack even basic knowledge of both compassion and the disease process.

There is no explanation for why my family was legally allowed to be torn apart and reassembled on the whim of a man, his attorney and uninformed court appointees, other than sheer ignorance. I mean the ignorance of not knowing, and by judging people harshly without proper consideration and information, because in the family court, you are guilty until proven innocent.

Despite being able to prove that I had never caused child abuse to occur, the lies that had been told about me, combined with my so-called odd behaviors, added to the suspicions of everyone around me.

Unfortunately, there was very little I could do to protect myself. The only persons who understood who I really was, were few and far between and even my many attorneys were unable to communicate exactly what was happening to me; other than the fact that I was "sick".

My ex-husband, when he set about to destroy my good name, did so with a vengeance. His comments to the psychiatric hospital intake coordinator did much damage to me and they affected how I was perceived by everyone involved in my daughter's very personal events.

He reiterated his earlier claims of my supposed mental illness to the school administrators, who chose to believe him. After all, no reasonably intelligent or normal person would make such serious allegations if they were not true, right? When I met with the administrative staff personally to discuss whether or not my daughter should be expelled from school, my ex had already convinced them, (in his meeting with them just hours before), that I was unstable and not to validate anything that I told them.

As a result, our meeting was tense, one-sided and uncomfortably short. I had the distinct feeling that everyone in attendance was merely humoring me and my husband. I only learned why much later on, and it was due to the things that my ex had alleged about me–my supposed mental problems. He had even dragged his post-divorce attorney into the meeting with the school officials, in an effort to garner any information that he could utilize against me at our next court hearing. His attorney was privileged with information that even I, as a parent to my own child, was not allowed to receive from the school. Now my ex and his attorney were out to get me through allegations of mental illness caused by Lyme disease, and they would stop at nothing in order to validate them.

These were the same two people who had originally openly mocked me in court, when I claimed that I was physically ill. They ridiculed my letters sent by my doctors, that verified that I had an undiagnosed illness, years before. My letter from an endocrinologist referring me to Mayo clinic was accused of being fraudulently acquired, and I believe because of that, it was subsequently inadmissable in court as evidence. When I did have a physician give phone testimony about a letter he had written that verified that I was unable to work, it did very little to help validate my health situation, because at the time even he could not provide the court with a medical diagnosis for me.

In fact, requiring the doctor to provide phone testimony completely alienated him from me as my doctor. After the court testimony, he fired me as a patient, citing that he no longer wanted to be involved in my family court problems. This was the second time I would lose a physician because of the on-going family court matters.

The court turned a blind eye toward me and my health situation, whether I had a diagnosis or not; choosing instead to find me guilty of a crime, the crime of being unable to work due to an imaginary illness; allegations that were currently on the table because of my ex-husband.

As the paper trail grew longer, the ability to defend myself from the allegations became much more difficult. Now my ex had even some of my family members thinking that I had mental problems.

My ex carefully listed my estranged mother and one of my brothers on his "witness" list, allegedly so that they could testify against me about my mental health issues and parenting abilities. Despite being related to me, these individuals had not seen me for between six and ten years, and their presence on his list was wholly inappropriate, if even known to them at all.

In 2005, after I had received intravenous treatment for Lyme disease and was feeling much more human than I had felt in years; I filed a motion to reverse physical placement of my children and rescue them from the hands of their father.

Both children had suffered cruelly because of the court's lack of vision in our case. My daughter had gone into a deep depression in part from her situation, but I believe in a greater part, from her illness. Most of the symptoms that she expressed in her over 900 separate internet postings are direct manifestations of Lyme depression and its associated mental changes.

My son was acting out behaviorally in school and at home. His grades which had been straight-A's when he lived with me, quickly slid downwards into the D and F range. Report cards showed comments like "not applying himself" and "disruptive" and "not up to his ability" on a regular basis. I knew that he was unhappy in his father's home, as was his sister, but both children had trouble standing up to their father's oppressive behaviors. He was hostile towards them and any signs that they might show any favoritism toward their mother.

The overtly bad behaviors that my son exhibited for three years now, were a reflection of both the external environment in which he lived and the internal physical environment within his body in which the Lyme spirochete flourished.

My ex worked overtime once my motion was filed, to again try to convince the children that they needed to make a choice to live with him. He threatened them (again) with moving far away from them and refusing to see them. He attempted to once again bribe my children with promises of shopping excursions and money. He purchased every kind of electronic game system on the market, in duplicate, so the children would have whatever gizmos they wanted.

He manipulated our seventeen-year old depressed daughter's thinking so much so that she actually believed that I was only "out to win" custody of her brother and that I no longer cared about her or what happened to her. She wanted desperately to run away from her situation at home and get away from both of her parents; though I submit that I did not play the same type of games that my ex-husband had done. In fact I did not play any games at all, I had merely spent the last several years struggling physically to be well and from being forced to repeatedly defend myself in court over his fabricated allegations of child abuse and mental illness that absolutely did not exist.

At one point after my daughter and I discussed her school emergency detention and how it had come about, she revealed to me that her father had told her that it had been *my* decision to put her into the mental hospital. When I showed her proof that I had no prior knowledge of the situation, for a brief period of time she had actually believed me, and things were going well between us. She finally believed that her physical (and mental) symptoms were actually a manifestation of her untreated Lyme disease.

My child dutifully took her medication as I directed her, and saw an improvement of her symptoms, that is until her father discovered she was taking medicine and took it away from her. He did the same thing with our son, refusing to allow me to treat their Lyme. When I sent him information about Lyme disease and the effects of it on the body, he ripped up the paperwork along with the Western Blot results and the doctor's diagnosis and chastized me for forcing them into my "delusions" of illness. I even felt the responsibility to inform him that Lyme may be sexually transmitted and to go and get himself tested. He laughed it off and declined to do so. At least I told him, others may not have been that magnanimous, considering our situation.

A parent with a vendetta and a strong will can well poison the mind of the brightest children thrown into a sea of confusion. He managed for a time, to convince both of the children that not only was I mentally ill, but that they were *not* sick with Lyme disease and that I was making that up in order to control them.

Even if I wanted to treat their Lyme disease right now, they refuse to talk about it and become very belligerent. They have heard enough of the squabbling over them, with me claiming that they are sick, and their father claiming "no they are not." Because of his refusal to grant me credence, they no longer want to be in the middle of the argument, sick or well.

As a result, I pray that they will not suffer many of the symptoms that I and others like myself have had to endure at the hands of Lyme. As I watch them slowly deteriorate however, I feel remorse that there was no way possible that I could have obtained a diagnosis for them any earlier than I did.

How sad and unnecessary that because their father refuses to validate me or his children's illness, that they will not receive necessary treatment while Lyme continues to affect their bodies in a negative manner; possibly causing long-term, irreversible damage.

Since I have filed a court motion to reverse physical placement of the children, my daughter is preparing to turn eighteen, and become an adult in the eyes of the court. She is planning to go away to college, and hopefully put some of her past behind her. In some respects I have to hand it to her, she has managed to keep her grades in high honor roll status throughout everything that she has experienced, and all while not feeling well during the process. But the damage to her and her brother is already done, and it will take years to reverse the emotional harm that our custody problems, and indeed our shared illness, has caused. I hope that as the children mature, I can convince them to undergo treatment for Lyme disease, and that they may one day, become truly well.

Our son on the other hand, at age fifteen, is still caught in the battle between what is right for him physically and emotionally and what my ex-husband wants to do to me, by using our son as an unwitting pawn.

The court, despite seeing us within its halls over the years, still has not managed to catch on to my ex's behavioral problems, and continually views me with contempt and a suspicious eye thanks to the negative paper trail he and his attorney have worked so hard to create.

My ex has now filed a counter-motion for sole custody and remove any of my remaining parental rights due to my "continual meddling" (read parenting) in my children's lives. He is attempting to do this by claiming that I (now) have a mental illness. Furthermore, that my "mental illness" is caused by my Lyme disease; the same disease that he and his attorney claimed I had lied about, only a few years before.

Ever since we proved the diagnosis of Lyme two years ago, they were forced to accept that I was indeed ill. But now they are attempting to exploit that very same illness and label me as mentally ill, with Lyme as a causative factor, to keep the children not only living with him, but also to remove my ability to parent by any legal means that remains.

His dispicable determination to shut me out of my parenting role by any means has stopped nothing short of driven. He has refused to allow me to speak with my children on the telephone, refuses to talk to me about any matters that concern them, and just plain refuses to communicate with me in any manner.

I have no clue what is happening in my children's lives except that which I can extricate from them or their schools, usually after the fact. I cannot participate in any decision-making processes no matter how insignificant, and I have to "let go and let God" now, where my children are concerned, because my ex does everything in his power to keep every aspect of their lives hidden from me.

Among many other things, he has managed to manipulate the

visitation schedule to his whims for many years and lies to me about the children's schedule, so that he can deny me my visitation time. He routinely appears late for visitation so that I am cheated out of more time with my children, all of which I patiently tolerate, because I refuse to play his games.

He tells the children lies about me and my motivations and fabricates whatever he needs to, to fit the situation at hand. He fabricates letters in court, lies on the witness stand, and tells lies to my family, to people who don't even know me, and to our children, about me. In case you are wondering, children always report a parent's bad behavior to the other parent—even if I don't really want to hear it.

My son is now much more protective of me, as he is reaching the age of maturity and is having his eyes opened to the antics of his father. And yet he is still caught in the middle, having three more years of the court's poor judgement in reversing our custody arrangements and he feels powerless to do anything about it. His continual regret at having originally lied to the court officers due to pressures from his father only adds to his feelings of anger and depression. He has had to struggle with his anger, and at times that has been very difficult with which to deal, in part because of the inner turmoil caused by court and his father's manipulations, and in part because of his physical symptoms of Lyme disease attacking his brain.

The battle unfortunately rages on to prove that not only do I *not have a mental illness*, but that the experiences our children have been put through at the hands of their father, have been *extremely harmful to them*. Even when I have attempted to live with the consequences of the court's poor decision-making, my ex-husband has continued to denegrate me, to no end, and filing motion after motion in family court in an effort to bankrupt both our finances and my credibility.

After seeing my children deteriorate from happy, somewhat

healthy children into sick, depressed individuals who seem to have no hope for a healthy future, I had to make the difficult decision to fight back.

I absolutely could care less really, what my ex-husband does to me or says about me. He has spent a good deal of the last decade, and an unbelievable amount of money attempting to tear our children away from me, at any price. The damage that his anger has done to his own family is irreparable, and yet the love that I have for my children remains, and I refuse to allow him to destroy those precious bonds, no matter what he and the court decide.

I know that whatever happens in court that it will be a very short time before both children are independent adults. And it is my hope that with maturity they will find a new clarity about our situation and their past. I maintain my connection with them on any level possible, no matter how small, constrained by the court or my ex's anger management problems, because I know that their future is yet ahead of them, and it includes their mother, and the love that I have for them.

I feel sorry for their father, for the most part, because he does not recognize that the seeds of the hatred that he has sown towards me (and is sowing) are going to blossom into regret. His own children that he claims to love so much, are not going to want to have anything to do with him before much longer. They are going to resent him for what they have been put through, just as my daughter right now blames me for the results of her recent actions. I merely discovered and brought them to light, because I love her and want to protect her from more serious consequences that she could have, and probably would have, faced. When she matures enough to reflect on her past, she will realize just how much I have done to protect her out of my genuine love for her.

Perhaps I will be lucky enough to finally show the court just how devious and destructive this man has been to his family. Perhaps I may even prove that I am not mentally ill, but that my only crime has been to be exposed to Lyme disease; an illness not only misunderstood by the court, but mired within its own controversy. Maybe I will convince the children, their father and everyone in the courts that my children have Lyme disease and that they need to be treated, **now**. (Well, one can always hope.)

For now, I have to work hard to continue within the court processes that I find myself, either voluntarily or through no fault of my own. And I must fight the most recent countermotion claims that I have a mental illness due to Lyme disease. On top of that, I have to continue to work toward my own personal wellness and get myself out from under the powerful grip that is chronic Lyme disease.

Last year after my daughter's stint in the hospital, my ex made the unfounded accusations that I was mentally ill. Attempting to ward off any of his claims the next time we had to appear in court, I voluntarily submitted to what would become, I believe, my third psychological profile since our divorce. The profile as expected, was quite healthy I am delighted to say, and was performed by a licensed doctor who was objective and previously unknown to me.

Although I don't really want to, nor do I have the money to actively pursue our current court motion, I have to plod along and do it anyway, for the benefit of my son, who is still miserably caught in the middle; partly for the benefit of both children so they have their medical issues addressed; and partly I admit, because I want to finally clear my good name.

My husband and I already filed bankruptcy due to the enormous costs of years within the legal system, and the huge medical bills that are left over from all my operations, doctor visits and recent Lyme treatments. Insurance did not cover much of any of those costs, and we found ourselves drowning in a sea of debt, with bankruptcy as our only way out.

Once we filed bankruptcy for our nearly two hundred thousand dollars in court and medical bills, some relief was immediately apparent, but now we live paycheck to paycheck in an effort to resolve our court conflicts and allow me to continue to receive proper medical treatment.

The tests for coinfections alone are prohibitively expensive, often costing hundreds of dollars per test. It has taken us many months just to be able to afford them, as they are not covered by our medical insurance. Many times already I have been forced to choose between receiving treatment for my disease or paying our attorney fees. That choice is one I (nor anyone else) should ever be forced to make.

My ex-husband now claims in court that we have all kinds of money and is actively trying to find new and clever ways to get his hands on our single income, as I still cannot work due to my ongoing illness.

He even ran down to the disability office the day he discovered that I had applied for it, in order to ensure that he was directly paid the children's benefits–a very generous eight hundred dollars per month. While I had already scheduled a phone interview to be their payee because I could not physically drive down to the social security office myself, he ignored this and took advantage of my situation and filed for benefits in person.

His doing this made him the payee, because he beat me to the punch, filing his paperwork first, even though I am the one who is disabled. I found his behavior particularly reprehensible because in court my attorney had distinctly advised him that I had already applied for benefits and not to do exactly what he had gone and done.

Just because I had my appointment scheduled but not yet completed, he decided he would slip in under the wire and grab ahold of the children's cash before I had a chance to complete the application process. Actually I really don't care who receives the money (if he was a normal person), but as you can well imagine, they have not seen one dime of that money, and somehow I doubt if they ever will.

Yes, with treatment I am physically better, significantly better than I was at this time last year, and I have come such a long way, but I still have a long way to go. I cannot drive very far, I still cannot eat food like a normal person. I am plagued with sleep disorders, occasional OCD, (counting), and mood swings. I have problems with balance and coordination, and strength issues, particularly on my left side. I do not seem aware of where my body is in relation to space, and I fall and receive other injuries frequently because of this. I require several naps during the daytime and it is extremely difficult for me to type at a computer, due to my vision which at best, is unreliable.

I often hear ringing in my ears, deal with painful insect-bite feelings and sharp stabbing pains in my skin. My joints, bones and muscles are painfully stiff every day and sometimes my headaches are so bad they approach migraine capacity. My vision fluctuates like the wind.

I am still on disability because I cannot yet support myself, and though I have tried to find work at home, I have been unable to do so in any meaningful capacity as I cannot put in even a half-day of work without difficulty.

I cannot arise before eight o'clock in the morning because my body simply does not function well, nor does my brain. If I don't sleep as long as I require, I get incredibly irritable and I fight with everyone around me. So sleep is imperative at this point, and not an option. I have long since ceased having hallucinations, and I no longer trash telephones, or throw objects, nor do I fly into fits of anger at small provocations. I genuinely laugh at the antics of my ridiculous ex-husband and work hard to eliminate the stress in my life as much as possible.

I still have sensory issues, brain fog and occasional problems with clarity of thinking, though I am much improved over where I was a year ago. I fully believe that with continued treatment I will improve, perhaps even to the point where I can become a

175

fully functioning adult in the world once more.

I struggle to maintain my balance whenever news of a negative nature concerning our court battle makes its way from my attorney's lips to my ears. I am not perfect, but I think I handle myself pretty well, considering all that we have been put through to date.

But I admit to having a few moments of difficulty remaining calm when my attorney contacted me following a recent status hearing. I was ordered by the judge to once again, sign medical record release forms so that my ex and his attorney could dumpster-dive back into my medical records. They are searching for a new clue now, any evidence at all, that they might find in their quest to defraud me in our upcoming trial. They want to prove unequivocally that I have some type of mental illness, so my ex can keep placement of our children, status quo. I think I mentioned that he wants to also remove any of my remaining rights for custodial parenting.

My ex and his attorney were *again* successful asking the court to allow them to harrass me by digging into my private files, under the assumption that I might have some mental health issues that need to be exposed. In addition, they have had the court order me to undergo my *fourth* psychological examination, designed to detect if I am mentally ill. This will mean more than eight hours of interviews with two forensic psychologists, including several hours of standardized testing, hopefully at their expense, all to inconvenience me as much as possible or worse, hopefully to try to provoke me into being belligerant so that I fail the examinations–and be labeled with some imaginary mental illness or personality disorder.

It was apparently not good enough that I had already done this kind of exam on my own accord and at my own expense to the cost of fourteen hundred dollars just a few short months ago. The court feels it necessary to allow the opposing side to force me to be evaluated by *their* psychologist, who is supposedly objective and independent.

A new custody study has been ordered (our fourth one in nine years), and the results of the psychological examination are also to be reviewed by the new custody evaluator, who knows nothing about our previous case history or the motivations behind the upcoming psychiatric evaluation.

I have no real rights whatsoever as far as I can tell, all because my ex-husband wants to claim that I am mentally ill in an effort to hold onto placement of our children, and probably, also the money he has coming in from my disability.

His lack of proof of mental illness and inability to validate this claim will prove to be his downfall. In the end, his decision will likely lead to him paying a very high price for his claims. If not in the courtroom, then certainly by the judgement his children render toward him for attempting to destroy their relationship with their mother, whom they love and will always love. No amount of effort on my ex-husband's part will ever tear apart those bonds, and I take comfort in that fact.

At the very worst I am inconvenienced yet again by having to drive four hours round-trip to the psychologist's office on two separate days, and then spend many hours being tested and interviewed. This will be very hard on me as I cannot travel great distances. I become very fatigued and there are other problems. Since I also cannot eat normally, I have to bring enough food with me in order to make it through the day.

I am sure that this "behavior" and my need to take breaks during testing for mental rest will not be reflected on in a positive manner, but I will do the very best that I can under the circumstances. And I think I will make a concerted effort to tell the evaluator that this is my fourth one of these examinations that I have had, with the previous ones describing no mental illness of any kind, just in case it makes any difference to the process. Perhaps I will provide him a copy of this book, which will clearly outline both the struggles my family has endured at the hands of my ex-husband and the family court, and most importantly, by virtue of having Lyme disease.

At best, the results of the test will prove once and for all that I have no mental illness. Despite whatever my ex and his attorney will try to claim, the evidence of all the psychological examinations over the course of nine years will clearly show that I am not impaired by my illness in a manner that would prevent me from being an exceptional parent.

However, just the mere fact that I find myself *again*, on trial due to *more* false allegations, this time of mental illness, and this time utilizing an illness that is as poorly understood as Lyme disease, irks me to the core of my being.

There is no place for disease in the family court system, unless it physically prevents someone from performing parenting duties, and in that case, should be objectively and carefully considered by experts before making a discriminatory judgement against a parent that would enable the reversal of previously ordered custody arrangements.

One might argue that if I *had* mental illness, that it could cause my parenting role to be reversed, perhaps appropriately. However, in my case, there has never been any evidence of mental illness of any kind, not even as "caused" by Lyme.

Despite that fact, the ability of my ex to file false allegations of both child abuse and mental illness that are unsupported with any evidence at all is what I am outlining here. The court *must* change its processes and force parents making these types of claims to *prove* those claims in the documentation submitted to the court *before* the court burdens itself (and families) with another custody case. This would prevent the types of situations my family found itself thrust into, for many years, at the hands of my misguided ex-husband.

In my opinion, **in the case where parents submit false allegations of child abuse against the other parent, and those**

allegations are proven to be false or wholly unsubstantiated, the court should punish the accusers severely, perhaps even with jail time.

This practice of accountability would certainly stave off many future antics of wrongly motivated non-custodial parents like my ex-husband (and their attorneys); and ultimately, save the innocent children who are caught in the middle of those struggles, from debilitating stress.

For children who are alleged to have an illness, especially one as *serious as Lyme disease,* **my wish is that the court fascilitate the ability of a non-placement parent to provide proper medical treatment for those children,** *especially* **when that treatment is in the best interests of the children, and when you have a situation** (like ours), **where one parent is attempting to block their treatment despite a valid diagnosis.**

It will take months for our court case to get to a new trial and I do not know what the outcome will be. I do know that in all likelihood, at least in the court's eyes, if my attorney does his job, than the erroneous claims of mental illness caused by Lyme disease that are alleged against me (and perhaps future parents) will be silenced, once and for all.   ❖

Follows is the full text (some names omitted) of the latest supposedly legal "medical release authorization forms" drafted by my ex-husband's attorney. The forms are intended for his utilization to obtain any and all of my personal medical files and information.

Please note that the authorization forms:

1.) remove any federal or state rights or protections to any of my records that "standard" authorization forms might provide, including protecting this attorney from any punishable improper use offenses;

2.) intend to reveal my private medical records to a medical provider whom I have never met nor spoken to, and who is probably not a Lyme-literate physician;

3.) allow the attorney to re-disclose my information to anyone whom he sees fit at any time and under any circumstances (unless revoked but that revocation does not apply to information already obtained);

4.) pretend to represent my personal wishes but do not;

5.) indicate that the order is voluntary when in fact I am under court-order to sign some kind of authorization forms.

The intent of the attorney is to obtain as much of my medical information as he deems fit, and then have it privately evaluated by a contracted mental health professional in his malicious attempts to try to fabricate a mental illness diagnosis and argue in court that his client should retain custody and physical placement of our children due to any diagnosis they wish to fabricate.

An important point I'd like to make in case it has not been made clear in this book, is that there has never been any diagnosis of mental illness in any of my medical files, nor has there been any discussion or exhibition of symptoms of same. But that is not the most important point here. I am suggesting that I have *no rights* and *no choice* by this attorney's document, should I be forced to sign same. I am being refused my basic rights provided at both the state and federal level–or I face contempt of court and face jail time!

Within my medical records, the varied misdiagnoses of my many physicians who are inadequately educated about Lyme disease and its symptoms will likely play a significant role in this evaluation process, which could tip the scales of justice in any direction.

Despite my medical records having plenty of wrong information within them, (and this can be argued), my ex's attorney will have his evaluator present a "professional" diagnosis of my mental health, by relying heavily upon these very medical records.

I have many questions:

1.) why am I not allowed to sign a "proper" medical release form from the medical providers themselves, which offers me at the very basic level, state and federal privacy protection;

2.) why must I be forced to forfeit those rights when I know that the intent to obtain the information is going to be utilized maliciously against me?

[Note: That malicious intent is punishable–there are civil and criminal penalties for violations of privacy. [15]*Generally speaking, penalties are assessed where organizations or individuals act with willful neglect or intent to cause harm. The criminal penalties for wrongful disclosure can include up to 10 years of imprisonment and $250,000 fines if used with the intent to sell, transfer or use for commercial advantage,* **personal gain, or malicious harm.** – EXACTLY WHAT THE ATTORNEY IS TRYING TO DO WITH MY RECORDS!

And I am supposed to waive my rights to protect <u>them</u> from punishment for allowing them to doing this to me.]

3.) why *would* I sign or *want* to sign such an authorization form, especially when it specifically *asks me to lie* (as stated in the document under section 9, paragraphs 3 & 4), that my signature is *voluntary* and that the document *reflects my wishes* when indeed neither one is true. **Am I supposed to lie to the courts just to placate them in order to affect such a release? Indeed, what would you do in my position? And moreover, why is this even a question?**

4.) The form allows the attorney to re-disclose my information as he sees fit and fails to identify by what means it will be re-disclosed.

By the way dear readers, while I do not have to disclose this information to you, I will for the purposes of this chapter. I have no history of alcohol or drug use, HIV or other sexually transmitted diseases, nor mental health issues. I am not attempting to hide some blockbusting personal or medical secrets that I feel threatens me in any manner, either.

What is the issue here is that I am being *required* to waive my **rights to privacy** and disclose my medical records in this form, and it **fails to allow me even the most basic state or federally protected rights to medical privacy.**

The issues of medical privacy rights are under their own controversy at present. I am not opening that can of worms, but I am trying to raise awareness of the abuse in the lower courts that is allowed to occur by wayward attorneys and uninformed judges!

Here is the authorization form in its entirety, excluding the omitted personally identifiable information and italics commentary within brackets, added by the author. Some bolded areas and spelling or grammatical errors originated within the document. The signature lines have been removed due to space limitations.

AUTHORIZATION FOR DISCLOSURE OF HEALTH INFORMATION

Patient Name: PAULA LANGHOFF
Date of Birth: xxxxx xx xxxx

1. I authorize the disclosure of the above-named individual's health information as described below.

2. The following individual(s) or organization(s) are authorized to make the disclosure: xxxxxxxxxxxx
[the names of the doctors' facilities entered here]

3. The type of information to be disclosed is as follows: All records; Referral Sheet; Discharge Summary; Clinical Professional Notes; Discharge instructions; Lab Results; Follow up Assessment/OASIS/60 Summary; Plan of Treatment; Medication Profile; Orally speak with the parties referenced in paragraph 5, above.
[I can tell you right now that my doctors are going to REFUSE to speak with this attorney, especially my Lyme doctor. Physicians want no part in either disclosing their patients' private medical records nor the courts–subpoena or not.]

4. I understand that the information in my health record may include information relating to sexually transmitted disease, acquired immunodeficiency syndrome (AIDS), or human immun-

odeficiency virus (HIV) (Act 148 Section 7 (e)). It may also include information about behavioral or mental health services, and treatment for alcohol and drug abuse (Section 7100.133).

[My Aids status? They are looking for __any__ excuse to withhold my paternal rights! Is that even legal?]

5. The information identified above may be disclosed to the following individuals(s) and/or Organization(s): Attorney (my ex's attorney of record and his physical address); Dr. (the name of the supposedly objective mental health professional who is being hired by my ex's attorney to examine my medical records) and/or (the name of his business, including staff, and physical address).

[I have no idea who this doctor is nor his qualifications nor his staff's, but I can guess his upcoming role in our court case will be to negatively evaluate and scrutinize my medical files and provide a "diagnosis" of my supposed mental health status, even though he has never met me nor examined me, nor does he, in all likelihood, have any accurate knowledge about Lyme disease.]

6. This information for which I am authorizing disclosure will be used for the following purpose: **Pending Post Divorce action: Langhoff vs. Lucas, Walworth County Circuit Court Case No. 97-FA-136.**

7. I understand that I have a right to revoke this authorization at any time. I understand that if I revoke this authorization, I must do so in writing and present my written revocation to the health information management department. I understand that the revocation will not apply to information that has already been released in response to this authorization. I understand that the revocation will not apply to my insurance company when the law provides my insurer with the right to contest a claim under my policy.

[Note, even if revoked, the revocation is completely ineffective against information already obtained, so what difference

would a revocation make; and why do the insurance compa-
nies retain their rights, but I do not?]

8. This Authorization is good until the following date: _____
If no date is specified, this Authorization will expire one (1) year
from the date signed.

9. Federal and Wisconsin Confidentiality laws protect this information. Such laws prohibit the re-disclosure of such information
unless further disclosure is expressly permitted by written consent
of the person to whom it pertains or as otherwise permitted by such
laws. However, I understand that the information disclosed may
potentially be re-disclosed by the recipient and may no longer be
protected by the federal privacy and confidentiality rules.
    [Note they acknowledge they are removing my rights.]

I have had an opportunity to review and understand the content of
this Authorization. I understand that this Authorization is voluntary.

I understand that I have the right to revoke this authorization at
any time. I can do so by submitting my revocation in writing to
the Medical Records Department. I understand that my revocation
will not apply to information that has already been released in
response to this Authorization.

By signing this Authorization, I am confirming that it accurately
reflects my wishes. A photocopy or facsimile of this Authorization
is as valid as the original.

Are they serious – You bet ya!   ❖

*"Whatsoever things I see or hear concerning the life of men, in
my attendance on the sick or even apart therefrom, which ought
not be noised abroad, I will keep silence thereon, counting such
things to be as sacred secrets."*
                    –Oath of Hippocrates, 4th Century BC

❖ Chapter 12 ❖

The Singing Forest

When I lived in the rental house in Fort Atkinson, my long nights staring out into the moonlit forest were the inspiration for a greater spiritual awakening. I already had so much turmoil within my life due to my illness and the struggles within the court system. I spent a lot of hours reflecting on the choices I had made in my lifetime and evaluated the path that I was on, both where I had come from, and where I planned on yet going.

I knew that my life had a greater purpose, as all of our lives do, but I had yet to discover exactly what that purpose was going to be. I struggled to make sense of my life, my family troubles and also to deal with the ongoing physical problems that I had.

When I experienced the singing forest, it leant me a serenity that I had not felt in a very long time. I began to look at my life from a higher perspective, one of appreciation for the simpler things in life, and the importance of valuing the gifts that are all around us, every day. No longer did I take for granted my time with my children, my health situation, nor anything else for that matter. I viewed people and their character flaws from a new angle also, one that understood that we were all people going through things in our lives, and that we were all essentially, students of life. I found a new value in those who motivated us to be better persons by virtue of their misgivings and (like my ex-husband), anger and foolishness.

My desire to make sense out of my life motivated me to search for answers. I read many books on medicine in order to find an answer for my physical ills. I researched the paranormal due to some of my hallucinations that were caused by Lyme disease. I studied spirituality and many religions for an explanation as to why human beings had to go through such negativity in order to live on this planet. Many of my questions received answers, and many did not; nevertheless my search continued.

When I finally was diagnosed with Lyme disease, I did not make a conscious decision right away to do anything except try to find someone who could treat me and make me well again.

I already had significant difficulty obtaining a doctor, and I knew of only one Lyme support group that might possibly recommend one for me. Unfortunately, the support group leader hesitated to do so, and openly asked me a huge number of questions designed to determine whether or not I truly was a Lyme patient. In the end I could not get any doctor referrals from the support group, which was not very supportive at all.

Not only was I unfamiliar with the disease state itself except for what little I had managed to read over the years, I actually had no idea yet just how steeped in controversy my disease was. Over time, my dismay would grow as I discovered that for years, patients with Lyme disease have been denied both a diagnosis and treatment, for a myriad of seemingly political and other reasons.

Because I had so much trouble getting help for myself, I decided that founding a support group in my regional area would be a good place to start. I had a twenty-six year background in publications, printing and design and nearly two decades of that included working with the internet and web design. So I fashioned both a web site and a Yahoo support group for Lyme and set about finding as much information as I possibly could to help promote the education of Lyme disease. In the process, I learned much more about the disease than I ever could have imagined I would learn or even wanted to know.

I named the web site www.Sewill.org, which represented Southeastern Wisconsin and Illinois Lyme Leagues. The site is pronounced "so-ill", because quite frankly, *we are all, just that.*

The site caught on and before I knew it, I had over a hundred members from my regional area, asking me for more information and links to web sites pertaining to Lyme disease and its co-infections.

Over the next year I began to network with other Lyme organizations and support groups and discovered both the grass roots and non-profit activities to raise awareness of Lyme disease. The subject matter was an incredibly tough nut to crack, as politically charged with as much opposition as it currently is.

I was sad and angry to see that there was literally no legislation in place that I could find, to protect doctors and their patients from state epidemiologists and medical boards and other entities who might attempt to quash physician's rights to treat their patients. Since then of course, Rhode Island has become the first to enact that kind of legislation, and I say **Bravo** for their courage.

I don't pretend to know the entire political history about how Lyme disease is handled in any arena, either medically, legislatively or otherwise, but I think I have sufficient information to be considered somewhat knowledgeable about both the controversy and the disease process.

In the last year I have been able to more clearly see the movement forming across the country that is attempting to erradicate the misinformation and discrimination surrounding Lyme disease, and that movement has originated from within the very least of its ranks, *its patients.*

Lyme patients from all walks of life are standing up, taking control of their illness and making a difference in this vast arena and are moving a piece of that mountain every single day. They are paving the way for Lyme patients like myself, and others yet in the future who will get this disease, the fastest growing vector-borne illness in the country.

I think I can speak for many of us in saying that it is our hope that no one else has to suffer the indignities of the kinds of things that early Lyme patients have suffered. If we can keep one patient, and hopefully all future patients from suffering either physically, mentally, emotionally, financially or discriminatorily, then I feel certain that we will have collectively done our job.

In the months that followed after the beginning of my support group, I was dumbfounded to hear of the stories that many Lyme patients had gone through. Many of them had been as bad as, or worse off, than I had been, and some had even committed suicide or have lost their fight against the effects of this insidious illness.

Most like me, had been unable to obtain a diagnosis for years, and were flat-broke, without adequate insurance or any insurance at all. Many treatments are cost-prohibitive, especially IV treatments, leaving many patients without any treatment options at all, if they can actually *find* a doctor willing or able to treat them.

All over the country, and indeed the world, Lyme patients are suffering needlessly, senselessly and horribly. In fact, if you have Lyme and live in Hawaii, you have two options. Either you travel to the mainland for treatment, or you live with the consequences of the disease. Like Hawaii, many states in fact have *no Lyme-literate physicians* at all, a term used within the Lyme community to describe doctors who have received adequate training in order to diagnose and treat Lyme patients properly. **These are not the "30-day and out" doctors that patients frequently encounter.**

One constant theme that I heard from the support group members and other Lyme patients was that they felt somehow "invisible". Family and friends did not understand what they were going through, and each one described how, like myself at one point, they felt as if they were losing their mind, and not in a mental illness-type way either.

To be able to relate to others on such an intimate level is a privilege and a blessing to me, and one that I don't take lightly. It is a huge responsibility when another human being trusts someone that they don't know, with such personal information. I am grateful for the trust and respect of each patient and story that comes to me.

Since I have so much "free time" according to my ex-husband, I one day took it upon myself to register yet another web domain name. I did not know exactly what I was going to do with it yet, but its name stuck in my head. Perhaps it was just the result of my creative juices flowing that day, but I registered **www.LymeLeague.com** and thought it might be helpful to have a site with that name at a future point in time.

That desire was finally granted about fourteen months later. As I read yet another story sent to me by a despondent Lyme patient, I got the idea that a web site was needed as a place for all Lyme patients to tell their stories. *There could be, and should be one place on the internet where all of our stories could be read, and finally, understood by everyone visiting.*

Perhaps patients, families, doctors, legislators, insurance and disability reps could go to that web site and see that we were **real people** dealing with **real disease**. Through the patients' own stories, I dreamed that my tiny web site could help eliminate some of the misinformation about Lyme disease, and lead others to a greater understanding of what the patient was experiencing.

I had already noticed one, or two, or even ten personal stories about Lyme disease on various support group web sites, but these were few and far between, and there seemed to be no singularly united forum for Lyme patients to get together and tell it like it is—in their own words, about their illness.

With no delusions of grandeur, I thought what the heck, I'm not doing much of anything right now, let's see if I can put something together. I thought I'd put it out there on a couple of support groups and perhaps acquire one, or two, or ten of my own stories for others to review.

The tiny web site was designed with the best of intentions. I struggled to create something that could be utilized effectively, in between the breaks I gave my hands and eyes, as I was having a hard time seeing what I was doing. My eyesight was a mess, but

I persevered anyway. I felt certain that my idea would be well-received; besides, I really needed something to do to take my mind off all the problems I was facing with the court matters.

In short, in about a week's time I had the site up and running on the internet, and within a very short time, I was innundated with responses from people all over the country, including from Canada.

Within a month, I had networked with a number of people and had many conversations with like-minded people, all fighting for the same cause. I was now fully thrown into the Lyme arena, much like one of those tiny insects I had encountered from the singing forest.

Since my diagnosis, I had already been sending information to every doctor I met who refused to acknowledge Lyme disease, especially chronic Lyme. But eventually, I became involved in the political portion of trying to help educate our Congresspersons about the plight of Lyme victims in this country.

I recently met with my district's Representative at one of his face-to-face citizen days, and discussed my experiences at length with him. I provided him with information designed to inform him about Lyme disease and the need for good legislation in order to protect both the physicians and their patients. I also told him about my Lyme support group and web sites, and much to my surprise, he and a few other legislators had already been to the newest site, www.Lyme League.com.

Other Lyme support group leaders from our state of Wisconsin are meeting with Senators and Representatives to the same end, and we collectively work as a team on a legislative committee of sorts. All across the nation, patients, support groups, non-profits and celebrities are lobbying Congressmembers to affect federal legislation and increase funding for the appropriate handling of Lyme disease at all levels, and end the suffocating misinformation and discrimination surrounding Lyme patients and their physicians.

As I write this book, right now in Congress there is legislation pending that would help provide $100 million dollars ($20 million over 5 years) for the research of Lyme disease. In the Senate is the **"Lyme and Tick-Borne Disease Prevention, Education, and Research Act of 2005", (S. 1479 Christopher Dodd/ Rick Santorum). The House companion bill, (H.R. 3427 Chris Smith/Sue Kelly)** is also up for consideration this session.

The bills are designed to improve surveillance and prevention of Lyme disease; develop accurate tests and fund research to study treatment modalities and effectiveness for long-term illness. They will also establish a Tick-borne advisory committee to ensure inter-agency coordination and communication among federal agencies, medical professionals, patients and patient advocates.

As an individual, you can help change the laws by contacting your Congresspersons at http://www.visi.com/juan/congress and saying you support this and other Lyme disease legislation.

While I do not know how the voting will go or if these important pieces of legislation will be accepted this time around, it is my hope and the hopes of many people in the Lyme community, that our government will act wisely and adopt these and future bills to begin the healing process for all Lyme patients.

In the meantime, it is up to each and every Lyme patient to stand up and be counted, as one singularly united voice. Do not accept doctors ignorance and being told that your illness is all in your head. Do not tolerate discrimination in the workplace just because you have an illness that is poorly understood or not yet protected.

Do not let the family court system take away your children from you just because it doesn't understand that there are illnesses that can make a person function erratically or poorly on the stand, yet still be an excellent parent.

Do not let an ex-spouse, together with his or her attorney,

manipulate the family court system into believing you have a mental illness just because Lyme or any other disease takes away your ability to think clearly or behave rationally once or twice, as in my case.

Make an effort to reach out to other Lyme patients in the community and teach people about Lyme disease *before* they become a victim. And for those already affected by Lyme, *be* the hand that reaches through the darkness that is Lyme disease, and guide your fellow human beings to a safer, more healthy place by whatever means you have at your disposal. There is no reason for a lack of support, and there is no excuse for ignorance about Lyme disease. The research is there, the patients are here, right in front of us, and *together we grow stronger.*

The medical community *must learn* that it is far better to be compassionate than to ridicule us and sweep their patients under the rug. The long-term costs to medicine are in the billions annually, and the numbers will keep increasing. Eventually, those in medicine will realize that it is **cheaper to heal us than to ignore us**.

Lyme patients and their families *must* band together to move this mountain of discrimination out of the way, one family at a time. We must change the laws to protect the patients and our doctors, so we can become well, whole members of society once again.

People in the medical community, social security offices, insurance companies and the community at large must become better educated about Lyme disease and the extent that this disease and its co-infections, can and do destroy lives. By allowing discrimination to prevail, we are allowing the erosion and elimination of our basic human rights. The right to privacy, the right to have whole families, the right for a diagnosis, and the right to become well.

By banding together, we will no longer feel invisible. By posting our names and stories to a site like **www.LymeLeague.com,** we can finally feel free to say that we *are visible.*

As we spread the word of this web site and our disease, people can read real patient stories and come to a new understanding of that which we have endured, lending dignity and meaning to all of our struggles, and indeed our lives.

The lessons that we can teach from our patient stories are all important, and each one of us can be like one of the tiny insects from the *Singing Forest*. As we sing our song of healing Lyme disease through unity and one voice, it is my hope that the music created will comfort all who hear it, and raise awareness of Lyme way into the treetops, and into the highest institutions of our government and medical community. ❖

– Peace and healing to all Lyme patients and their families,

PJ

"Truth passes through three stages. First, it is ridiculed.
Second, it is violently opposed.
Third, it is accepted as being self-evident."

– *Arthur Schopenhauer (1788-1860)*

❖ Chapter 13 ❖

After Words

I feel it necessary to speak here a bit about IV treatments, which are steeped in controversy. In my case, after surveying some of his patients, I learned that my doctor treated all of his patients with a single, standard protocol. We were all given the exact same doses and mixtures of medications, irrespective of our body type, weight, or infections, and that was probably not the best method possible for us. It is my opinion that the *methodology* used to treat me via IV was inappropriate in my case, and *not* the IV treatments themselves or the types of drugs that were used.

Still, I am a very good example of how **IV treatment for Lyme disease is absolutely and directly responsible for pulling me back from the brink of permanent disability.** I am unbelievably grateful that I had that opportunity, however short or difficult, when I had it. I know that without those treatments, I would have fallen into the abyss that is Lyme disease; and my health would have been irretrievably lost as a result.

IV treatments for Lyme disease, I believe, when administered properly and in the right doses, are a life-saving option for chronic Lyme sufferers. In my opinion, from personal experience, and yes from so-called "anecdotal stories" from other Lyme patients, especially those who have been misdiagnosed for so long, (like me), they are absolutely critical.

While I am not completely well yet, I am substantially better and am working with my doctors on treatment options that are now orally-based, and which are working to slowly erradicate the various infections present in my body. I also do what I can to eliminate toxins, take supplements and perform strenuous reconditioning exercises, which is absolutely essential in order to achieving total recovery.

I have watched myself unable to walk across a room or lift a milk carton gain back the strength and ability to perform basic horseback riding several times a week. This ability took many months of exhausting work to achieve, but I have done so, nevertheless. Last year at this time I would have thought it only a dream to be able to recover that much of my function.

It is my hope that by 2007 I will be well enough to return to work and cast off disability for good through proper antibiotic treatment. Hopefully my children will, at some future point in time, also have both the opportunity and the ability to get the treatment they deserve, so that they too can continue on their life's journey, but as whole persons, and free of Lyme disease.

Many of my co-infections, have been eliminated by the various antibiotics I received over the years, and yet Lyme and some remaining co-infections persist inside of me.

I cannot stress enough how important it is that Lyme patients have proper diagnosis and treatment in Lyme's earliest stages, before the devastation that it causes, translates into years of needless suffering and expense to its victims.

It is my firm belief that the events in the lives of my family would have taken an entirely different course if only Lyme disease had been properly diagnosed and treated at its onset, fourteen years ago.

Doctors can do better, and patients *deserve* better. Doctors, listen to your patients. Patients, become educated about your disease and treatment options. And to everyone else, I would like to say please become educated about the *prevention* of Lyme disease and related illnesses, your life may just depend upon it.

Support your family members who contract Lyme disease, and get involved in their treatment process. We are *real* people, living with *real* disease and we have the need for respect and compassion. We as Lyme patients have the desire to become well; we have that *right* and we deserve that *chance.* ❖

❖ Chapter 14 ❖

Lyme Links

⏎Visit these important web sites for more information about Lyme disease:

- The Lyme Disease Association
  PO Box 1438, Jackson, NJ 08527
  Email: LYMELITER@aol.com

  www.lymediseaseassociation.org
  888-366-6611 information line
  732-938-7215 fax

- The Lyme Disease Foundation, Inc.
  PO Box 332, Tolland, CT 06084
  Email: info@lyme.org

  www.lyme.org
  800-886-LYME (5963) 24-hr.
  860-870-0070 phone
  860-870-0080 fax

- The Lyme Disease Network of New Jersey
  43 Winton Rd., East Brunswick, NJ 08816

  www.lymenet.org
  support & discussion

- California Lyme Disease Association
  CALDA, PO Box 707,
  Weaverville, CA 96093

  www.lymedisease.org
  Email: info@lymedisease.org

- ILADS (International Lyme and Associated Diseases Society)
  PO Box 341461
  Bethesda, MD 20827
  Email: lymedocs@aol.com

  www.ilads.org
  301-263-1080 phone
  301-263-0776 fax

- Canadian Lyme Disease Foundation
  2495 Reece Rd., Westbank
  BC V4T 1N1
  Email: jimwilson@telus.net

  www.canlyme.com
  250-768-0978 phone
  250-768-0946 fax

- WILDER Network
  (World International Lyme Disease Emergency Rescue Network)
  P.O. Box 116, Forestville, CA 95436
  Email: WILDERnetDRAGON@wildernetwork.org

  www.wildernetwork.org

Lyme Links, continued

* Diagnostic Hints and Treatment Guidelines for Lyme and Other Tick-borne Illnesses, By Joseph J. Burrascano, Jr., M.D.
www.lymediseaseassociation.org/burrguide.html

* Yahoo On-line Lyme Support Groups: http://health.dir.groups.yahoo.com/dir/Health___ Wellness/Support/Illnesses/Lyme_Disease
(yes, those are 3 underscores, but no spaces between them, in the address line)

* Lyme League of America
PO Box 444, Hustisford, WI 53034
920-349-3855 phone
Email: pjay@lymeleague.com

www.lymeleague.com

The place to tell your personal story about Lyme Disease!

* Dr. James L. Schaller
Community Bank Towers,
Newgate Ctr., Suite 305
5150 Tamiami Trail, N.
Naples, FL 34103
239-263-0133 phone

www.personalconsult.com
Office Suites Plus
7320 E. Fletcher Ave.
Tampa, FL 33637
813-909-8009 phone

Dr. Schaller is currently working on books about Pediatric Lyme, Bartonella and Babesia. His own extended family was nearly destroyed by Lyme. He offers extensive free Lyme education material at his web site, listed above.

& Such

The author highly recommends these publications for more information about Lyme Disease and its co-infections:

Coping with Lyme Disease, 3rd ed., by Denise Lang,
ISBN:0-8050-7563-1; Available at major book sellers

Lyme Disease Update: Science, Policy & Law
Includes insurance, disability & workers' comp info.
ISBN: 0-9758776-0-7; www.lymediseaseassociation.org

Confronting Lyme Disease, What Patient Stories Teach Us
by Karen P. Yerges and Rita L. Stanley, PhD.
Intimately portrays the struggles of Lyme patients.
ISBN: 978-9764384-1-0; www.confrontinglyme.com

Lyme in Rhyme by Geri Rodda, R.N.,
illustrated by Jillian Zampaglione
Delightful children's educational book explaining Lyme Disease in
Rhyme; Available at: nmroddas@aol.com

You Don't Look Sick! Living Well with Invisible Chronic Illness
by Joy H. Selak, Steven S. Overman
ISBN: 0-7890-2448-9; Available at major book sellers

The Lyme Times, PO Box 707, Weaverville, CA 96093-0707
Subscribe for informative issues covering testing, current lyme issues,
pediatrics and lyme and much more! www.lymetimes.org

Another book by PJ Langhoff:
Right Behind You, Spiritual Helpers From Beyond the Earth Plane
A fascinating look into the possibility that our lives are more than just
a biological happenstance, or accident of nature.
Theme: alternative/spirituality. ISBN: 978-1-4116-8443-0
Available at: www.lulu.com/content/248718 and major book sellers

"Do not live in a town
that has no doctors."

– *Old Jewish Proverb*

❖ Bibliography ❖

[1,16]Information provided by P. Mervine, CALDA; as taken from publicly-funded studies, and from the Legislative packet for support group leaders.

[2]Excerpts from the Center for Disease Control's web site as published on April 12, 2006. (www.cdc.org)

[3]Center for Disease Control web site under the topic: *Case Definitions for Infectious Conditions Under Public Health Surveillance,* dated March 2006 and includes case definitions for 1995-1996. (http://www.cdc.gov/epo/dphsi/casedef/ lyme_disease_1995.htm)

[4]*Coping with Lyme Disease, 3rd ed.* by Denise Lang, ©2004, Henry Holt & Company, LLC

[5]Excerpts from the *MMWR Morbidity and Mortality Weekly Report, Surveillance for Lyme Disease, United States, 1992-1998;* by Kathleen A. Orloski, D.V.M., M.S. et al. and updated April 28, 2000, 49(SS03); 1-11, (http://www.cdc.gov/mmwr/preview/mmwrhtml/ss4903a1.htm)

[6]Census Bureau's web site as published 04-12-06, (http://www.census.gov/popest/ estimates.php)

[7]*MMWR Morbidity and Mortality Weekly Report, Surveillance for Lyme Disease, United States, 1992-1998;* by Kathleen A. Orloski, D.V.M., M.S. et al. updated April 28, 2000, 49(SS03); 1-11, (http://www.cdc.gov/mmwr/preview/m mwrhtml/ss4903a1.htm)

[8]From the E-Medicine web site, *Lyme Disease,* by Julie L Puotinen, PharmD, Clinical Coordinator of Pharmaceutical Services, et al. (www.emedi- cine.com/neuro/topic521.htm, update 11/28/05).

[9]The Wisconsin Department of Health & Family Services web site; *Health Disease Fact Sheet Series, Lyme Disease",* (http://dhfs.wisconsin.gov/communicable/ communicable/factsheets/LymeDisease.htm as of 04/06)

[10]The CDC's *Data Warehouse report, GMWK I Worktable,* Total deaths for each cause by 5-year age groups, United States, 2002, p. 142.

[11,12]From IDSA's *Guidelines for Lyme Disease,* Wormser et. al., CID 2000;31 Suppl 1, p. S3.

[13]Lyme Times, Summer 2004, volumes 37 & 38; published by The California Lyme Disease Association (CALDA)

[14]From "Klebold paper foretold deadly rampage" by Holly Kurtz, *Denver Rocky Mountain News,* Nov. 22, 2000

[15]From "Medical Privacy", on the Electronic Privacy Information Center, www.epic.org/privacy/medical

Printed in the United States
83034LV00004B/158/A